Clinical Cases in Dermatology

Series Editor
Robert A. Norman

Tien V. Nguyen • Jillian W. Wong
John Koo

Clinical Cases
in Psychocutaneous
Disease

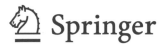

Tien V. Nguyen, MD
Department of Dermatology
University of New Mexico
Albuquerque, NM
USA

John Koo, MD
Department of Dermatology
University of California
San Francisco, CA
USA

Jillian W. Wong, MD
Department of Dermatology
University of California, Davis
Sacramento, CA
USA

ISBN 978-1-4471-4311-6   ISBN 978-1-4471-4312-3   (eBook)
DOI 10.1007/978-1-4471-4312-3
Springer London Heidelberg New York Dordrecht

Library of Congress Control Number: 2013951351

Printed on acid-free paper

Springer is part of Springer Science+Business Media (www.springer.com)

Preface

The Dilemma

Competency in communication and interpersonal skills is a core requirement of the Accreditation Counsel for Graduate Medical Education. One can make the argument that our formal medical education system leaves something to be desired regarding this aspect of patient care. Studies have shown that effective interpersonal communication on the part of the practitioner can have a powerful effect on the patient's satisfaction with his/her dermatologic care, can possibly improve treatment compliance and health outcomes for the patient, and can decrease the likelihood of malpractice claims against the practitioner [1–6]. Unlike basic clinical skills, such as obtaining a history of illness or performing a physical exam, communication and interpersonal skills can be more difficult to teach and to assess. As such, even experienced clinical instructors may be at a loss regarding how to impart these skills, in spite of their best intentions to help the trainees communicate more effectively with patients.

Two common challenges in dermatology can hinder effective practitioner-patient communication and patient education. One, we are constantly under the time pressure created by short visits, and as a result, our patients sometimes leave the visit with the impression that they were rushed by their dermatology practitioners. Two, the heavy focus on youthful, flawless skin in modern society has influenced many of our patients to develop unrealistic expectations in terms of the extent to which therapy can completely clear their skin diseases. These challenges contribute to the mounting stress of demonstrating effective interpersonal communication on the part of the practitioner, especially in situations involving difficult patients (e.g., those with a long problem list, unrealistic expectations, unusual demands, etc.).

A Patient-Centered Approach to Resolve the Practitioner-Patient Interpersonal Issues

In addition to basic training at the undergraduate and graduate medical education levels, communication and interpersonal skills necessary for establishing therapeutic rapport (i.e., a trusting relationship) with difficult patients can be acquired and polished with experience in practicing medicine. We recommend supplementing your knowledge of this topic by continually seeking outside educational resources, including didactic seminars taught by healthcare communication experts as well as books and other publications. It might also be helpful to reach out to any colleagues, including but not limited to psychologists, psychiatrists, and medical anthropologists – they are well-versed on topics pertaining to interpersonal relationships in the medical setting.

The following seven scenarios represent what appear to be the most common cases in dealing with difficult patients, ranging from the "long list" patient and the patient with a chronic disease to the distrustful/poorly compliant patient. We also grouped the cases according to specific elements of the visit (i.e., agenda setting, expectation management, apology and trust building), to help you identify areas needing development. With this section of the book, the authors hope to achieve two objectives: (1) to advance understanding of the psychological and social nuances of a dermatologic visit with a difficult patient, and (2) to help the readership develop useful techniques to resolve any communication-related issues. Even though the cases that we have created for this book are hypothetical, we hope that the teaching points will provide you with some helpful insights and practical knowledge, as they were derived not only from the authors' experiences in dealing with difficult patients but also from those of our respected colleagues.

Of note, the concept of patient-centered care (i.e., where the patient is at the center of any healthcare professional-patient relationship) is at the center of our philosophy about how to approach difficult patient cases. We hope that you will take the care to listen and consider all of the possible factors causing certain patients to appear "difficult" – from obvious to subtle to even hidden factors. The authors believe that great lessons can be learned from this humble approach to human interactions. Our reflections on the emotional reactions that the difficult patient may evoke in each of us can lead to an expanded understanding of ourselves. How can we learn better ways of giving advice? Are we fully aware of the emotional impact on the patient's psychological state of heart-felt expressions, such as "I wish I could make this better for you" and "I wish this weren't happening to you"? Do we know when to say nothing except "I'm Sorry"?

As the first part of this book is a learning experience for all of us, your input is welcome at the lead author's email address, letien62nguyen@gmail.com. Thank you in advance for your help.

Albuquerque, NM, USA   Tien V. Nguyen, MD
Sacramento, CA, USA   Jillian W. Wong, MD
San Francisco, CA, USA   John Koo, MD

Series Preface for Springer Clinical Case Reports Books

It is my great honor to be the series editor for the Springer Collection of Dermatology Case Reports Books. The case report format is a wonderful tradition and is particularly important in today's rapid-fire times.

Proposed Series Books will include Geriatric Dermatology, Inflammatory Disorders, Sexually Transmitted Diseases, Integrative Dermatology, Atopic Dermatitis, Dermatological Surgery, Wound Care, Malignant and Benign Neoplasms, Bullous Diseases, Hair and Nail Disorders, and other important subjects. Each book of didactic cases is of great practical help to both experienced and novice dermatologists. Although each book's primary audience is dermatologists, it can also provide guidance to internists, family physicians and emergency room doctors.

I believe that each book in this series will greatly contribute to the education of those that carefully study and read the cases. My great hope is that the patients of every practitioner that has absorbed and applied the lessons in each of these books will benefit from these case studies.

I have worked with Grant Weston and the staff of Springer for many years and I know they produce consistently excellent books and have a wide distribution and international readership. Thanks to Grant and all the Springer people for their hard work and energy.

Thank you to all the wonderful authors for their insight, time, and determination to bring each book to fruition. Each of these books reflects the contribution that these talented authors and editors have made to add more light to the art of medicine and the care of our patients.

Dr. Rob Norman

Acknowledgements

The authors would like to thank Steve Shama, M.D., for his tremendous help with reviewing and editing this book.

Contents

xvi   Contents

Abbreviations

BDD	Body dysmorphic disorder
DoP	Delusion of parasitosis
DSM-IV	Diagnostic and Statistical Manual of Mental Disorders-IV
FDA	Food and Drug Administration
MDE	Major depressive episode
MHP	Monosymptomatic hypochondriacal psychosis
OCD	Obsessive-compulsive disorder
PCP	Primary care physician
PTSD	Post-traumatic stress disorder
SDI	Spectrum of delusional ideation
SSRI	Selective serotonin reuptake inhibitor
TCA	Tricyclic anti-depressant

Part I
Psychologically Challenging Patient Encounters in Dermatology

Chapter 1
The "Long List" Patient

Dr: Hello Mr. Hawthorne. How are you today?

Pt: I'm good, Doctor. I brought a list with me so that I don't forget to ask you anything before I leave. Can we go down the list starting from the top?

Dr: Thank you for bringing in the list. I see that you have marked all of these 15 items as important. Do you want to talk about all of them today?

Pt: Yes, please. It's so hard getting an appointment to see you. I want to have all of my concerns addressed so that I don't have to wait until next time.

Reflections on the Case

Patients are often asked by their practitioners and the practitioner's medical society to create a list so as to have all of their concerns resolved in the most efficient way possible. The problem with Mr. Hawthorne' list is its length, causing you to worry about being able to address them fully and comfortably in a single visit. It is important to take a step back and explicitly acknowledge that this patient has been proactive about taking care of his health. This well-intentioned effort on Mr. Hawthorne's part and the ultimate product, the list, are not meant to purposefully control the visit or create unreasonable demands on your time – but to save time during a seemingly

T.V. Nguyen et al., *Clinical Cases in Psychocutaneous Disease*, 3
Clinical Cases in Dermatology,
DOI 10.1007/978-1-4471-4312-3_1, © Springer-Verlag London 2014

short dermatologic visit. Of note, there might be other possible explanations for a patient's list, including insurance reimbursement issues and conflicts with the patient's personal or work schedule, etc. Therefore, it is important to wait until the patient finishes his opening statements in order to find out his motivation for making a long list.

Teaching Points

When it is your turn to speak, the authors suggest beginning with: "Mr. Hawthorne, thank you for taking the time to make this thorough list." Patients like to be complimented by their practitioners for doing something good, and here is your opportunity to gain favor with Mr. Hawthorne, even though you might feel apprehensive about the list's length. Second, ask politely to look at the items on the list with him, keeping in mind that he most likely expects you to have an infinite amount of time to address all of his concerns in a single visit.

A useful intention on your part would be to assume that Mr. Hawthorne composed his list in innocence, not realizing that some signs or symptoms may require lengthy conversations and exams. In order to make the patient more amenable to shortening the list, remind him gently: "Mr. Hawthorne, I would love to spend time addressing each item on your list in a careful, thorough manner. However, if I were to do that, it would take up more time than what I have scheduled for you today. I understand that you might not have realized this before. Would it be okay if we look at the list and choose the three most pressing concerns to take care of in this visit?"

If the patient was successfully persuaded to shorten the list, consider yourself lucky! However, the authors of this book are less optimistic about this happening with the average "long list" patient. Therefore, we will prepare you for the case where Mr. Hawthorne does not agree to accept your request. You can start the argument for a shorter list by saying, "I'm afraid that if we completely evaluate all of your concerns today, we will not be able to focus on the most important problems requiring a lot more time and attention than the others. In addition, if we address every item on your list, I might overwhelm you with too much information. I'm sorry."

Occasionally patients might not accept the above explanation and continue to insist that you deal with every item on the list, even if this means information overload. Some practitioners employ the tactic of guilt-tripping patients by saying such things as, "I'm sorry that we cannot accommodate all of your needs today, Mr. Hawthorne. As you can see, there are other patients waiting outside to be helped. I cannot spend all of my clinic time with you today because it means that I would have little or no time to see those patients."

The authors are not sure of the success of this tactic. You are essentially setting boundaries with Mr. Hawthorne by saying "I do not have enough time to help you with all of your problems." Such an approach requires much experience and can backfire, resulting in an angry patient. Only you can determine whether or not it is worth possibly sacrificing a long-term relationship with a patient to stay on schedule, by limiting what you will and will not discuss from the list. Sometimes you might decide to acquiesce in the request of the "long list" patient so as to get through the visit and part on an amiable basis.

It might be helpful to reinforce your compassion for the patient by looking directly at him and saying in a warm tone, "Mr. Hawthorne, I understand that getting an appointment to see me is difficult. I would love to see you again and again, and take the time to get all of your skin problems under control. So if we cannot get to a couple of problems on the list today, I promise that we will take care of them promptly at the next visit. I am here for you!" You really have to mean what you say – Mr. Hawthorne expects you to follow your own words with strong actions.

If it is within your capacity, you may also suggest that a phone call be scheduled later that day or the next day to deal with non-urgent issues on the list. In our experience, given the opportunity to call, most patients do not embrace it.

However, it is reassuring and comforting for the patient to be offered such an option, and your chance of convincing these patients to shorten their lists might be made more favorable. Before ending the visit, it might be wise to go over the list again and show him that you took note of the items not addressed in this visit. Mr. Hawthorne may become more confident about your ability to deliver the high-quality, compassionate care that you promise him.

Chapter 2
The "Will You Be My PCP?" Patient

Ms. Bronte is a previously healthy 35 year-old woman, who presents to you as a new patient with sudden-onset generalized plaque-type psoriasis. She also complains of intermittent achy joints and a sensation of chest tightness that typically precedes each flare of psoriasis. She has received a thorough work-up from multiple specialists, including dermatology, rheumatology, and cardiology, at a respected medical institution prior to coming to you. In spite of having previously been diagnosed with psoriasis, she claims that her condition has not been fully diagnosed, and she worries about the risk of a cardiovascular event. Reports from cardiology and rheumatology revealed no obvious causes for her symptoms. The patient is sitting in front of you, appearing very anxious and distressed about her health, and pleads that you help control her psoriasis as well diagnose her heart and joint disease. In other words, she wants you to be her primary care physician (PCP).

T.V. Nguyen et al., *Clinical Cases in Psychocutaneous Disease,*   7
Clinical Cases in Dermatology,
DOI 10.1007/978-1-4471-4312-3_2, © Springer-Verlag London 2014

Reflections on the Case

As dermatologic practitioners we occasionally run into skin disorders associated with systemic diseases, and some patients might ask you to treat non-dermatologic manifestations of such diseases. Ideally, we wish we could be knowledgeable across all disciplines of medicine so as to be able to address all of our patients' concerns, both related to and not related to dermatology. But we may not be or feel that we are not adequately trained in other specialties, and often enough need to involve the help of our respected colleagues. Most patients do understand this limitation of our specialty, but unfortunately, not all of them do.

Teaching Points

For patients who confuse our role as a specialist with that of a primary care physician, such as our well-meaning patient Ms. Bronte, it is your responsibility to inform them that you are not able to diagnose and manage non-dermatologic disorders. "Ms. Bronte, thank you for sharing your concerns. I understand that you are very anxious to have all of your questions answered. May I point out that some of your concerns fall outside the scope of my specialty? I would love to help; however, for your benefits it might be best to involve your primary care practitioner in this process. If needed, he/she will be able to refer you to the appropriate experts in joint, heart, bones, etc. who have been trained to address issues related to these organs." Emphasizing the important role of her PCP is a good strategy, and you should follow it up with a reassuring statement: "I promise to work closely with your PCP to manage your overall health. We are a team."

The authors have observed that in some instances fear is the motivating factor for the "Will you be my PCP?" patient. If you ask Ms. Bronte why she wants you to take care of her heart and joint disease, she might reveal: "Doctor, I have so much faith I you. You helped one of my best friends when she had a serious skin condition. And recently, I have been worried having a heart attack. One of my girlfriends just passed away last month due to a heart attack. The day before, she seemed to be as healthy and happy as ever, and the next day she was gone…poof, just like that. It got me thinking: what if the same thing happens to me?"

In response to Ms. Bronte's heart-felt disclosure, it is appropriate to attempt to console and reassure her, with the understanding that her emotional distress might have played a big role in exaggerating her health concerns. You should also ask if she is amenable to seeing a psychotherapist for emotional support during the grieving process, since her friend's death is fairly recent. From your perspective, creating healthy outlets for her guilt and sadness can take some of the focus away from her exaggerated health concerns, specifically with regard to potentially life-threatening systemic diseases that have not been conclusively linked to her skin disorder.

The authors recognize that sometimes you need to say **no** to a patient. For instance, if Ms. Bronte insists that you replace her PCP for whatever reasons, you may decline such a request, unless of course you are truly comfortable with becoming her PCP. As a dermatology practitioner, you should maximize your empathy for patients when possible; however, we recommend against pushing yourself beyond your boundaries of expertise in order to be nice. It is best to establish your role and the boundaries of your responsibilities with all of your patients, especially those demanding services that you are not comfortable providing. The approach to the "Will you be my PCP?" patient is similar to that for the patient "long list" patient and the patient with unusual demands, where the overall goal is to skillfully set your boundaries without offending the patient.

Chapter 3
The Patient with Unusual Demands

Mr. Twain is a 46 year-old man with hidradenitis suppurativa that has not been active for the last year. At his last follow-up 3 months ago, he reported groin pain in spite of a benign physical exam. Today his chief concern is again pain: "Doctor, I have been aching in my armpits a lot recently. I haven't seen any boils and bumps in these areas, but I keep feeling the pain. It's worse at night when I try to go to sleep."

The physical exam is, as it was noted last time, unremarkable. You perform a thorough review of Mr. Twain's medical chart, paying close attention to his problem list and history of medication use. It appears that he has had a long history of chronic back and shoulder pain unresponsive to high doses of non-steroidal anti-inflammatory drugs, gabapentin, and morphine analogs. After you finish reviewing the chart, he states, "As you can see, I have tried many pain killers in the past, so I know which ones work for me. I want you to give me some hydromorphone to get rid of the pain in my armpits."

T.V. Nguyen et al., *Clinical Cases in Psychocutaneous Disease*, 11
Clinical Cases in Dermatology,
DOI 10.1007/978-1-4471-4312-3_3, © Springer-Verlag London 2014

Reflections on the Case

Patients can sometimes make seemingly unusual demands, some of which might be justifiable once you understand the motivation for such demands. They may be malingerers, drug seekers, or simply frustrated with the lack of improvement of their symptoms and/or how you are handling their care. Sometimes, possible culprits causing a patient to make surprising requests may be industry advertisement or strong recommendations of their friends/family. It behooves every practitioner to be patient and listen to the patient's narrative with an open mind, since any pre-conceived notions about the patient's motivation can cause you to listen selectively and as a result, miss important details about the patient's true motivation or concerns.

Mr. Twain might have an ulterior motive behind his request for hydromorphine, as the physical exam is inconsistent with his report of significant pain. Additionally, the fact that he is very specific about the type of pain medication he wants should raise another red flag. The authors have observed a number of different approaches to manage this situation. Some practitioners would give Mr. Twain the benefit of the doubt and prescribe him hydromorphone to reduce his armpit pain, in spite of the aforementioned red flags. Other practitioners might be wary of perpetuating possible drug dependency on the part of the patient, and thus take a more conservative approach than their counterparts when prescribing pain medication. We respect the reader's point of view on this controversial subject matter and the decision you ultimately make.

Teaching Points

If you truly believe that Mr. Twain is making an unreasonable demand, the next steps are, in temporal order, to explain why you cannot fulfill his wish, make an offer for what you can do now to lessen the pain, outline a plan of action, and most critically, ask for his approval of this plan. There are two objectives for the explanation you provide to the patient. First, be sure to make apparent your best wishes for his wellbeing: "Mr. Twain, I care about your wellbeing and understand how much the pain in your armpits is bothering you."

The second objective is to explain why you are not able to meet his demand, gently yet firmly: "I am sorry. However, based on my assessment of your disease I am not comfortable with writing you a prescription for hydromorphone. It has possible side effects and a tendency to cause patients to become addicted. In my opinion, at this point the risks might outweigh the benefits." Then, you might be able to lessen his disappointment by emphasizing the things you are able to do for him: "Mr. Twain, please remember that I do want to take good care of you. It appears that the pain you feel is associated with a deep, inflamed boil. I would like to give you a pain medicine called naproxen, which can also reduce the inflammation of the boil."

Finally, provide a plan of action with determination and enthusiasm, and ask for his approval of this plan: "I would like to for you to try naproxen for 2 weeks. If the pain does not get better in that period of time, I will be happy to consider prescribing a stronger medicine. By working together I know that we can get this problem taken care of. Does this plan sound okay to you, Mr. Twain?" Hopefully, the patient and you agree on the plan you have just outlined. If the patient still insists on getting what he wants, it is appropriate to give a firm no, keeping in mind that you have done your best given the circumstances. A referral for a second opinion may be offered at any time that you sense great resistance or anger from the patient.

Chapter 4
The Fearful Patient

Ms. Austin is a healthy 21 year-old woman, who appears very anxious in the waiting room. She has a 2-year history of acne vulgaris unresponsive to herbal remedies, topical retinoid agents, and combined topical antibiotic/benzoyl peroxide preparations. She reports that within the past 3 months she has suffered significant discomfort and public embarrassment from the inflamed deep cysts. She is here to get a second opinion about how to improve her acne, stating that her general practitioner has done everything in his power to help her.

Ms. Austin's past medical history is unremarkable, and she is currently not taking any medications. Physical exam reveals mixed severe inflammatory and moderate nodulocystic acne. Surprisingly, it appears that she has never been given oral antibiotics or oral retinoids. When you broach the subject of trying an oral antibiotic agent in combination with her topical regimen, her strong rejection of your recommendation takes you aback: "Is this a pill, Doctor? I don't want to take any pills because they are not good for my body. I have heard many horror stories about people having bad side effects while taking pills. These cysts are terrible, but they don't kill me – I would rather leave them alone than taking pills to make them disappear."

T.V. Nguyen et al., *Clinical Cases in Psychocutaneous Disease*, 15
Clinical Cases in Dermatology,
DOI 10.1007/978-1-4471-4312-3_4, © Springer-Verlag London 2014

Teaching Points

Ms. Austin reminds us that the same medical information can be perceived very differently from patient to patient. Some patients have no problems taking systemic medications despite clear warnings about significant yet rare adverse effects, while others are reluctant to take anything internally. It is the practitioner's responsibility to sort out the patient's fears so that the best approach to controlling her severe cystic acne is ultimately discussed. All of the basic communication and interpersonal skills (e.g., reflective listening, refraining from interrupting the patient, sitting instead of standing while talking to the patient, etc.) are key ingredients in developing a good relationship with a patient who might be fearful of possible adverse effects.

"Ms. Austin, would it be okay if I asked you what questions or concerns you have about this medicine? I promise to do my best to answer them." A few good things have been demonstrated in these sentences. First, you have shown respect by asking for permission to delve into her fears. Second, you have left an open space for the patient to fill in by phrasing your question as an open-ended request. "What questions or concerns you have" is preferred over asking, "Ms. Austin, do you have any concerns about this medication?" If she is ambivalent about verbalizing her concerns, a close-ended question can easily lead to her answering "no." Third, the simple phrase "I promise (*or* I will try) to do my best to answer them" is designed to make the patient feel reassured and comfortable with discussing issues that might have induced her emotional distress.

Similarly, if the fear is due to uncertainty about whether or not a medication will be therapeutic, then the optimal approach may involve providing reassurance and support. Of note, reassurance can be empty when you have not effectively conveyed that you share Ms. Austin's perspective. Simple things such as smiling, leaning your body toward the patient when she narrates, demonstrating empathic communication (i.e., naming the emotion she seems to be expressing, understanding, respecting, and supporting her feelings), are all powerful ways to achieve this goal. It may be appropriate to indicate that you have had experiences similar to Ms. Austin's current situation, without disclosing personal details (i.e., "What I am asking you to do might make you feel nervous. I know this because I have been a patient on a few occasions and got to see things from the other side."). Showing this patient that you are a vulnerable human being while still maintaining your professionalism (i.e., refraining from over-sharing) might actually help you develop a stronger bond with her.

In addition, it is common for patients to become fearful due to information they have learned that does not apply to their skin diseases. Thanks to the Internet, dermatologic patients can readily access any information available to the public at the click of a mouse. Unfortunately, there has not been any well-established Internet "filter" to help them navigate through this large well of information. Thus, you might have to provide some guidance for your patients in this regard. For instance, Ms. Austin might disclose, "I read on this blog by a young woman close to my age that she took some pill the doctor gave her for acne, and then her face swelled up like a balloon. That really freaked me out, Doctor." This has been termed "Google terror" by Dr. Neil Prose because the patient's fear is a result of her learning information that is erroneous, pertaining to extremely rare events, or non-applicable to her case.

In the hypothetical example above, the authors recommend not immediately rebuffing the likelihood of her face swelling up like a balloon, as this might make you appear dismissive to the patient. Please think of it as a legitimate concern. You should compliment Ms. Austin for having done her research on the skin disease: "I applaud you for spending time and effort to learn more about acne. It is often helpful to know that other people have similar experiences as you." After positively reinforcing her self-efficacy (i.e., the idea that the patient can do a lot to improve her condition), the next moment is a good opportunity to counter her negative impression of the medication, "Ms. Austin, what I am saying is based on my medical knowledge as well as personal experience prescribing these acne pills to many patients. It is very unlikely that your face will swell up like a balloon if you take them the way I ask you to. I understand your concern, but I don't think that we should worry about it right now."

According to Dr. Prose, one way to prevent "Google terror" is to anticipate what the patient will possibly find and warn her in advance: "Ms. Austin, you might run across something called acne inversa and descriptions of painful boils in the groin, armpits, or buttocks. This is not what you have, so if I may say this, please ignore it." This is a strategy to help the patient filter out inappropriate information on the Internet. As a result, she will likely be less anxious before and during subsequent visits, and you can focus your time and energy in those visits to address her legitimate concerns.

Chapter 5
The Patient with a Chronic Disease

Mr. Dickens is a principal at a local high school, who has been seeing you for the past 2 years about his chronic urticaria. He is typically a very pleasant and compliant patient. As an educator, Mr. Dickens values the patient education component of his visits with you, and is generally eager to share his experiences of living with a chronic skin condition. When he started with you, each urticarial episode lasted up to 12 h and occurred approximately every other day. Once aggressive therapy was instituted, his condition gradually improved to the point where he now experiences an episode every other week, with each one lasting no more than 1 h. Today is his regular 3-month follow-up, and the receptionist noted that he appeared quite unhappy.

Pt: Doctor, I had a bad flare yesterday. It took nearly 10 h to clear up.

Dr: I'm really sorry to hear that, Mr. Dickens. Did you do all of the things we had discussed to control this episode?

Pt: Yes, I did. I even took an extra anti-histamine pill just to see if that would help, but it didn't. I have been under a lot of stress lately, and I notice that each episode has lasted longer. Other than that, everything else in my life has been the same, including my treatment plan.

T.V. Nguyen et al., *Clinical Cases in Psychocutaneous Disease*, Clinical Cases in Dermatology, DOI 10.1007/978-1-4471-4312-3_5, © Springer-Verlag London 2014

Dr: Stress can play a big role. Have you tried relaxation techniques such as yoga or meditation? In terms of therapy, would it be okay to add another anti-itch pill to your current regimen for better control of the current breakthrough episodes?

Pt: I'm tired, Doctor. It has been about 3 years; yet, these breakthrough episodes have not completely gone away. My positive spirit can only carry me so far. When will they find a cure to help me get rid of my disease?

Reflections on the Case

The case of Mr. Dickens, who is living with a chronic dermatologic condition, illustrates how best to deal with patient expectation and satisfaction. Two things could be responsible for his unhappiness: (1) He expected highly effective therapies that can cure his chronic urticaria, whereas what you are able to provide is long-term maintenance of good disease control, with no guarantee of a cure, and (2) He is mentally exhausted from having to keep up with relapses occurring in an unpredictable fashion despite good compliance and adequate support from you. These expectations are typical of psoriasis and eczema patients as well as patients with chronic urticaria, and patients frequently ask their dermatologic practitioners to explain the fickle nature of the disease. Unfortunately, no simple evidence-based answer exists to satisfy the patient's thirst for knowledge in this regard.

A study by Uhlenhake et al. showed that most patients with psoriasis did not grasp the concept of maintenance therapy for their disease [7]. The study did not investigate how this failure on the part of the practitioner to educate patients impacted patient satisfaction and health outcomes. After reading this book, the authors hope that you will be more mindful about setting realistic expectations and helping your patients comprehend the merits of long-term mainte-nance therapy. This is not to say that they should abandon all hope for a cure.

Teaching Points

The most important step in trying to help Mr. Dickens is to understand what expectations he already has with respect to therapy for his chronic urticaria. You may ask, "Mr. Dickens, how would you like for me to help you?" This is best done at the beginning of your first visit; however, it is never too late and oftentimes necessary to re-assess his expectations, espe-cially when he voices dissatisfaction with care. It might also be helpful to tease out specific elements needing your atten-tion by asking, "Do you think that I could be doing more to help you, or are you simply frustrated that there is no cure for your condition? I am curious to know what other concerns you might have."

In many instances, a patient's unhappiness is a result of both his high expectations of the care you provide and his frustration with the chronic nature of the skin disease. Our practical approach to dealing with this situation consists of two components. One, explain clearly what he can expect in terms of the prognosis and treatment course. Two, provide realistic hope and emotional support for any psychological issues related to the disease. Regarding setting expectations, you may delineate a step-by-step treatment plan, "Mr. Dickens, here is what I am able to help you achieve. If you take both types of the anti-itch pills every day during the first month, then you might experience three episodes per week, and each one will likely become shorter and less itchy. The next month, continuing this regimen hopefully will lead to one episode per week, with each one lasting even shorter. After the third month, you might experience a very mild attack once every other week, with each one lasting maybe 1 h."

Having a chronic, unpredictable disease that seems to be out of the patient's control can be very frustrating for both you and him. As such, the more details you give in your explanation of the treatment plan, the better he will feel. Additionally, we encourage the use of empathetic and compassionate statements, such as "I can only imagine how troubled you must feel," or "Mr. Dickens, I am always here if you need any form of assistance or support regarding your disease. If I cannot help you, I promise to find you someone who can."

As a disclaimer, you should always state, "your individual progress might differ from this plan. However, I think that we can still get your disease under control. What I am not able to do is to offer you a cure. I only wish I could. To my best knowledge, no doctors or practitioners have a cure for chronic urticaria yet." Some practitioners like to drill the "no cure" concept into the patient's head before discussing available therapeutic options. The author (TN) has observed that patients tend to have an easier time accepting this prognosis if you explain the merits of disease control first, "Mr. Dickens, even though there is no cure for your disease, there are still things we can do to get it under control so that you can have most of your normal life back." Such an approach does not encourage false hope – it provides the much-needed reassurance to cushion the possible huge disappointment of learning that his condition is incurable at the present time.

To conclude the discussion of this case, the authors would like to emphasize the therapeutic effect of adequate emotional counseling to counter the patient's mental fatigue. Not infrequently, psychological stress related to other issues at work or at home can add to the stress of managing a chronic disease. It is critical to show your caring and enthusiastic attitude in providing **timely** support when the patient truly needs it; however, it is up to you to decide how to achieve this goal. Some practitioners give selected patients access to their email addresses or cell phone numbers.

This "VIP" (**V**ery **I**mportant **P**erson) treatment comes with one caveat that must be clearly communicated in order to void possible future issues: "Mr. Dickens, you already have my office phone number. If you need help with an urgent problem, please call my secretary first, and she will do everything in her power to help you. For some reason, if you need my attention immediately, you may email or call me. Would it okay if I asked that you use your best judgment when deciding whether or not to email or call me? Please know that I am here for you." In addition, you should determine if he needs additional counseling from a mental health professional, and be sure to ask for his permission before making a referral.

Chapter 6
The Angry Patient

Mr. Hemingway is 45-year-old business executive with a very busy work schedule. He was seen in your office yesterday morning for a concerning flat, uniformly brown mole that had been expanding from 3 to 8 mm in diameter and darkening for 6 months. A 3-mm punch biopsy of the lesion was performed, and you distinctly remember having placed the skin specimen in its properly labeled container before sending it to the pathology laboratory. This morning, you received a message from the administrative assistant in the lab stating that no specimen was found in the container for Mr. Hemingway. You called the manager of the lab and asked for help. Sadly, after an exhaustive search of the lab, Mr. Hemingway's specimen still could not be found. You also performed a similar search without finding the specimen.

You now call Mr. Hemingway directly to explain and apologize for the loss of his skin specimen. He sounds very upset, "Doctor, this is completely unacceptable. Do you have any idea how busy I am? I had to use up my lunch break and cancel an important meeting to be able to see you and have that procedure done. Now you're telling me that you are not able to find my skin specimen? What kind of a show are you guys running over there?"

T.V. Nguyen et al., *Clinical Cases in Psychocutaneous Disease*, 25
Clinical Cases in Dermatology,
DOI 10.1007/978-1-4471-4312-3_6, © Springer-Verlag London 2014

You attempted to mitigate his anger by offering to perform another biopsy free of charge at his earliest convenience. To this he responded, "No thank you. What if that specimen would have revealed skin cancer, and now it's lost? I am going to call my insurance company and ask them to get a refund for the procedure that you did yesterday. And then I will write a letter to the dermatology board to request an evaluation of your competency. Doc, rest assured that you will never see me in your office again."

Reflections on the Case

This is a very unfortunate event and possibly the result of someone else's mistake, whether in your office or in the laboratory. However, as Mr. Hemingway' care provider you are ultimately responsible for any concerns the medical error may cause; thus, his anger is directed at you with nowhere else for you to shift the blame. Such a case as this might even lead to serious medico-legal ramifications, since a diagnostic specimen has been lost. However, you could make a good argument to him that since the lesion was flat and uniform in color, a repeat biopsy of the lesion performed within a respectful time frame would be just as representative. While the issue is important to recognize, the concern of a malpractice suit is beyond the scope of this book. Good communication skills can reduce the likelihood of the patient considering the medico-legal path.

Our main goal is to help you develop effective communication skills to convey a heart-felt, sincere apology and hopefully be able to mitigate Mr. Hemingway's anger. In situations where there is an adverse event, patients typically want three issues addressed. They want to know the fact (i.e., how could this have happened?). They want an apology. And they want to know what you intend to do so that the same event will not happen to someone else. One thing to keep in mind is that anger can be an expression of a single or a combination of other emotions, including fear, anxiety, disappointment, and guilt, etc. For many patients, anger is typically a cry for help.

It behooves you to listen to Mr. Hemingway and understand where he is coming from. Is his current attitude really an expression of anger over a lost skin specimen and the inconvenience of a repeat biopsy, or is it a disguise for his fear of possibly being diagnosed with melanoma? There is no doubt that the process of waiting to hear the biopsy results can be very stressful for patients – might he be disappointed that no results are given and possibly be averse to going through this process again? Being able to understand and explicitly state your understanding of the patient's emotion can be tremendously helpful for conflict resolution with regard to adverse events. Please consider using the NURS approach previously discussed: **N**ame the emotion the patient is feeling (e.g., "You seem very upset"), **U**nderstanding (e.g., "I can truly understand why you would feel this way"), **R**especting (e.g., "I respect that you feel this way"), and **S**upporting the patient's emotion (e.g., "You have every reason to feel this way").

Teaching Points

When in the presence of an angry patient, it is important for you to always check your emotional response to any negative and/or provocative comments he might make. The authors suggest taking deep breaths to center and relax yourself before the encounter. During the encounter, if you sense that a looming conflict is unavoidable, sometimes it might be beneficial for you to leave the phone conversation or the examination room and find a quiet space to assess the current situation. Even if you think that Mr. Hemingway does not have a good reason to be upset with you, honoring the fact that he could be upset with you is important.

One way to set up for a more pleasant conversation with Mr. Hemingway and work toward mitigating his anger is through one or two genuine compliments to the patient at the beginning: "I hear your frustration loud and clear. If I may say, I can tell in the short time that we have known each other that you are a very nice person. I hope that you will allow me to explain what had happened to the best of my knowledge, and to offer you my apology." In terms of how to phrase the apology, you can say "I wish this had not happened to you" or "I wish there were something else we could have done to prevent this from happening to you." The two words "something else" indicate that you had done your best to prevent the loss of his skin specimen. These longer phrases also convey your best wishes for Mr. Hemingway' well-being and render the adverse event less as an issue of negligence on your part and more as a result of an innocent mistake.

If you are able to pacify his anger, the next crucial step is to follow your apology with an action plan outlining how you will investigate, follow up, and fix the root cause of the adverse event. Angry patients such as Mr. Hemingway are typically worried that the same error will happen to them again or to others in the future. As such, they would like to be reassured that permanent, systematic changes have been set in motion. Suggest a plan to him, and after you have explained it thoroughly, you might want to say, "Mr. Hemingway, does this sound like a reasonable plan to you?" And be sure to follow this up with "What other suggestions do you have for me at this point?"

The second open-ended question has a strategic purpose – by asking for Mr. Hemingway' opinions you have successfully expressed your view of the relationship with him as a work partnership. In medicine there has been a gradual departure from the traditional, paternalistic model of the practitioner-patient relationship, with more emphasis on developing "patient-centered care" (i.e., the patient is at the center of the relationship). As such, you can view the encounter with the angry patient as a unique opportunity to empower him and let him know that you have his best interests in mind. If you are not comfortable with this strategy (and we recognize that some of you might not), please respect our intention.

Finally, you have a solemn obligation to Mr. Hemingway to make sure that a re-biopsy is preformed, regardless of the outcome of your conversations with him (i.e., either you or a colleague that he may choose to see can perform the re-biopsy).

Chapter 7
The Distrustful and Poorly Compliant Patient

Ms. Dickinson is a 56 year-old new patient presenting with severe scalp dermatitis and psoriasiform scaling, for which a tentative diagnosis of scalp psoriasis has been made. She reports trying several topical agents, each for a few days on six different occasions over a 3-month period, with inadequate control. The referring dermatologist, who called you prior to the patient visit, is concerned that her insufficient response to therapy has been a result of poor compliance. He notes that she typically resists his treatment recommendations, and on several occasions has made blanket statements indicating her distrust of medical professionals.

During the visit, Ms. Dickinson appears indifferent to your smiling, sits with her arms and legs crossed, and avoids direct eye contact when you address her. Toward the end of the visit, you say: "I would like to prescribe a medication that comes as a liquid to get rid of the flakey, red spots on your scalp. Would you be willing to try this out for 4 weeks and then come back to see me? Does this sound like a reasonable plan?" She responds, "I am not sure, Doctor. People have given me many medicines for my scalp condition, but none of them helped. My last dermatologist promised me many things. In the end, he gave up on me. So why should I trust you?"

T.V. Nguyen et al., *Clinical Cases in Psychocutaneous Disease*, 29
Clinical Cases in Dermatology,
DOI 10.1007/978-1-4471-4312-3_7, © Springer-Verlag London 2014

Reflections on the Case

Gaining a patient's trust is fundamental to establishing a good relationship with that patient, especially when you know that the patient is distrustful and/or when you suspect that she is poorly compliant. Sometimes this is a difficult goal to achieve because not all patients appreciate what we can do for them nor how hard many of us work for them. In our litigious society, cases of malpractice claims against certain practitioners can become sensational. As a result, some patients might be influenced by such stories to view all medical professionals as threats as opposed to their allies.

In addition, some patients may form negative impressions of healthcare workers from published stories of medicine-related adverse events, or from their unpleasant experiences in the healthcare system. You might suspect that this is the case with Ms. Dickinson – one clue is the bitter tone with which she described her previous dermatologist. Whatever the true cause of her distrust is, she is now predisposed to poor or non-compliance, which can lead to poor treatment outcomes that will further undermine what little trust she has for you. The way that you communicate with Ms. Dickinson can have a positive impact on your relationship by promoting her to develop respect and confidence in your competency.

Teaching Points

First, you may make a gentle request for an explanation: "Ms. Dickinson, I would love to help you feel better by improving the condition of your skin. As such, it's very important that we understand and work closely with each other. Would you mind letting me know what specific reservations you have about my ability to help you?" You have addressed the issue head-on; yet, the words you have selected convey a desire to establish honest communication with her, and more importantly, a sense of caring. If anything, this caring attitude may have the effect of disarming Ms. Dickinson, who could have put up a barrier just to test if you truly care about her as a patient.

During the interview, Ms. Dickinson relates an important story that helps explain her distrust and poor compliance: "I used to listen to every word coming out of every doctor's mouth. My father is a doctor, and I grew up admiring what he does. It made me want to become a doctor, but I ended up choosing chemical engineering. Anyway, 2 years ago, I underwent an emergent procedure because my inflamed appendix had exploded. After the surgery, I still had a lot of stomach pain and felt as if I was still infected. It turned out that the surgeon had left a couple of dirty sponges inside my body. I realized then that doctors are not gods – you guys make honest, simple mistakes that can kill people like me. So again, why should I trust you?"

It would appear that Ms. Dickinson's distrust is a manifestation of her fear of a possible life-threatening adverse event. As such, it should not be viewed as a personal reflection on your clinical knowledge or interpersonal skills. One helpful strategy that some practitioners employ is to say, "Ms. Dickinson, I get it now. The experience that you had with the previous surgeon has left a scar in your mind about what doctors can and cannot do. I do my best – by listening to you, making the best diagnosis, suggesting the best and safest medications, checking that prescriptions have been properly written and dispensed, and checking back with you to make sure that you are getting better. Please keep in mind that I do care very much."

Here you have demonstrated a number of important points to build Ms. Dickinson' trust. You anticipated her safety concerns regarding the medication prescriptions and dispense. This should suggest to the patient that you can think from her perspective and are indeed a patient advocate. You also appease any uncertainty she might have about your competency by promising to check back with her and make sure that your recommendations are effective. This can be done via a phone or an email prior to the follow-up appointment. The authors understand that you might not have unlimited time and resources; however, in the context of a distrustful and poorly compliant patient, making an effort to perform this extra step can go a long way.

Finally, involving a distrustful patient in her care is an intelligent strategy, as it gives her more control and fosters a teamwork spirit with shared responsibilities and open communication. If you are not sure how to answer a question or address a concern Ms. Dickinson has, you may say: "I'm sorry, but I do not have an answer for you right now. Would it be ok if I called you later today so that we can have a more in-depth discussion of your question? I will try to provide you with my best answer then." When all of the processes about how you make decisions regarding diagnosis and treatment are transparent to Ms. Dickinson, she will be more likely to work together with you to become a trusting patient.

Part II
Psychocutaneous Disease in Geriatric Patients

Special Considerations for Geriatric Patients with Psychocutaneous Disease

Being aware of the growing presence and influence of the geriatric population in dermatology as well as psychodermatology is critical to a successful practice. One, the Baby Boomer generation, who now compose the majority of the elderly population in the United States, contribute significantly to the number of patient visits to dermatology practitioners. It is estimated that by 2020, approximately 25 % of the general population in the United States will consist of people aged 65 and older [8]. Other countries around the world, such as Japan, Germany, Greece, Italy, and Sweden, are also experiencing the same problem, with the elderly accounting for approximately 20 % of their general populations, respectively [9].

Two, understanding the unique challenges that elderly patients face can help you develop safer and more effective treatment plans for such patients. For example, important biomedical changes such as decreased cognitive impairment with age and physical disability should be taken into consideration, in addition to an increased dependency of geriatric patients on their caretakers for assistance with daily activities (e.g., finding transportation to a physician's office, being able to apply topical medications to areas of the skin that are difficult to reach, etc.). When systemic medications are indicated, you should review certain aspects of the patient's history with care, including co-morbidities, functional status of the drug metabolizing organs (e.g. liver and kidneys), and poly-pharmacy (i.e., the institution of multiple drugs taken on a daily basis, often for more than one disease), etc., to ensure maximal safety.

The following three cases represent common psychocutaneous conditions that a dermatology practitioner is most likely to encounter in the elderly population. Of note, one helpful clue to help you distinguish cutaneous manifestations of psychopathology from true dermatologic disease is the area of distribution: please pay attention to the locations of the skin lesions. If they are primarily concentrated in easily accessible areas, such as the extensor surfaces of the arms or the hands, the disease is possibly self-induced. The authors recognize that exceptions do exist, and as such, the importance of taking the patient's history meticulously and performing a thorough physical exam cannot be overstated.

Chapter 8
Delusions of Parasitosis in Geriatric Patients

Mrs. Jones is a 90-year-old Caucasian female, who was brought in to see you by her son for a 12-month history of chronic biting and stinging sensations all over her body. She had not observed any bugs to bite or sting her skin; however, the sensations she felt are those that could only be created by insects. As a result of being frequently bothered by these sensations, she repeatedly picked at her skin in places she was able to reach. She also reported retrieving several types of "materials" embedded in her skin. They often appeared as insect body parts and clear, coiled fibers, which she claimed "were shed from the bugs." She had brought some of these objects in plastic zip-lock bags to the dermatology clinic and requested you to examine them as carefully as possible.

Upon further questioning, the patient stated that the infestation had started during her long-term stay at an assisted living facility. After the patient made several complaints to the staff of the facility, extermination teams were hired to search for and exterminate the infestation. Yet, according to the reports of several different companies, no bugs of any kind were found in her room or anywhere else in her housing unit. Previously, three general practitioners had seen the patient in hope of eliminating the bug infestation. Again, none of these practitioners were able to find any ecto-parasites on her skin, and as such, they provided here with reassurance, which she did not accept. Your physical examination revealed multiple superficial excoriations with some scabbing, but no evidence of ecto-parasites.

Reflections on the Case

The most common psychocutaneous condition in the geriatric population is delusions of parasitosis (DoP) – with a documented sex ratio of 3:1 in favor of women [10]. Studies have reported the average age of onset among older adults to be 55.6–65 years [11, 12]. As illustrated by the case of Mrs. Jones, affected patients frequently have an elaborate, firm belief that they are chronically infested with living organisms (e.g., insects, parasites, etc.). These patients seek referrals to dermatology practitioners in hope of having their "skin lesions" examined, usually with scraping and microscopy, for evidence of body parts or fibers thought to belong to the infesting organisms. The primary goal they have for the visit with you can be validation of this fixed belief, which the authors also refer to as a delusional ideation. Most of these patients will also complain of formication sensations (i.e., crawling, biting, and stinging), and of course, will ask for your help to improve such sensations. However, depending on the degree of the delusion, seeking relief from these symptoms is not necessarily the most important goal of the patient.

Teaching Points

In order to avoid misdiagnosing the patient, the authors advise exhausting the possibility that Mrs. Jones' symptoms stem from an internal condition or a neurological process. She had seen multiple practitioners prior to you, and the following tests had been ordered and come back with negative results: hepatic enzymes, thyroid function levels, vitamin B12 level, creatinine, a complete blood count, and a basic electrolyte panel. If this had not been the case, you would need to order the aforementioned laboratory tests. In addition, a consult with neurology should be placed to rule out underlying neuropathology affecting cutaneous nerves, such as multiple sclerosis or a chronic cerebrovascular disease. Of note, elderly patients might have abnormal reactions to drugs thought to be safe in the general adult population; as such, please take the care to verify their medication history and check for adverse effects or drug interactions that can potentially cause delusional beliefs.

Once the diagnosis of DoP has been made, referral to a mental health professional may be indicated [13]. Please keep in mind that many patients with this condition refuse to see a psychiatrist or a psychologist because they do not believe that the underlying cause of their symptoms is of a psychiatric nature. Therefore, you need not push the issue regarding the referral and risk jeopardizing your relationship with them. Instead, try to be diplomatic and do what it takes to forge a therapeutic rapport with these patients first, and this might involve examining any specimens brought in by the patients under the microscope, as in the case of Mrs. Jones. If you do not find anything, it is okay to be honest with her, "I believe you. However, I am not able to find any parasites on you or in these specimens today." Saying "I believe you" with a sincere tone can possibly help the patient feel less invalidated and more connected with you.

After therapeutic rapport is established, you may carefully broach the topic of instituting pharmacotherapy with an antipsychotic agent called pimozide (Orap®) to improve symptoms of formication and hopefully reduce the delusional ideation [14]. Since potentially fatal arrhythmias have been reported in patients taking pimozide, you should order an electrocardiogram to assess for pre-existing arrhythmias or prolonged QT intervals. In terms of safety concerns specifically for the geriatric population, be sure to pay special attention to certain anti-cholinergic properties and extra-pyramidal effects of pimozide (e.g., drowsiness, stiffness, etc.) that may predispose elderly patients to an increased fall risk. The authors recommend clearly explaining possible adverse effects as well as preemptively forming strategies for the patients and their family/care-takers to manage such events.

Chapter 9
Neurotic Excoriations and the Elderly

Ms. Blackburn is an 83-year-old new patient, who presents with multiple lesions over her arms and legs. She relates a history of volunteering on and off for the past that she began volunteering at a community garden 6 weeks ago, and she has recently been bitten by ants. She states that the lesions from the ant bites have become progressively worse over the past few days. Her lesions have recently demonstrated crusting and weeping of yellow discharge. The patient has come to see the dermatologist because she is concerned about infection of the lesions. She also reports she has recently become very anxious and depressed, as her husband passed away 2 months ago. On physical examination, there are multiple excoriations over the extremities. In addition, during the interview, the patient constantly scratches at her arms and legs.

Reflections on the Case

Neurotic excoriations present as self-induced cutaneous lesions often caused by obsessive picking, scratching, rubbing, with or without pruritus being reported. Generally, patients have a strong desire to scratch combined with poor control over these impulses. Common psychiatric disorders associated with neurotic excoriations are anxiety, depression, and obsessive-compulsive disorder. Such behavior can also be related to social stressors. Neurotic excoriations most predominantly occur in women and the average age of onset is in the older adult population, specifically starting during the third to fifth decade [15–17].

A key to diagnosing this condition is the clinical distribution of excoriations. Excoriations often appear in areas that are easily accessible to the patient, such as the extensor arm and anterior thigh, while difficult to reach places, such as the bilateral upper, lateral back area, is typically spared. The "butterfly sign" is a characteristic feature, in which the areas of sparing where the patient cannot reach to scratch at the skin resembles the shape of butterfly wings [17]. The excoriations can become infected, as in this case.

A patient with neurotic excoriations should be worked up for medical and other psychiatric differential diagnoses. Medical causes for true skin itching leading to self-induced excoriations include cutaneous dysesthesia, malignancy, xerosis, hepatitis, urticaria, and uremia [18]. Psychiatric conditions leading to excoriations include anxiety, depression, obsessive compulsive disorder, dermatitis artefacta, delusions of parasitosis, dermatitis artefacta, hypochondriasis, and borderline personality disorder [14].

The first-line treatment depends on the underlying psychiatric diagnosis. For depression, selective serotonin reuptake inhibitors (SSRIs) are recommended [19–21]. For anxiety, anxiolytics such as benzodiazepines can be used with caution for the elderly patient. For pruritus, doxepin 5 % cream or menthol or phenol containing lotion with an emollient base may be prescribed. Extreme caution should be used when considering oral anti-histamines for pruritus in an elderly patient due to strong sedative and anti-cholinergic effects. Topical antibiotic agents such as mupirocin 2 % ointment or oral antibiotics such as cephalexin may be needed for infected cutaneous lesions.

Chapter 10
The Geriatric Patient with Neurodermatitis

Mrs. Hightower is a 79-year-old African-American female, who presents to the office with her husband with a chief complaint of persistent bug bites and edema of the lower extremities. The lesions in question are reported on both arms from the wrist to mid upper arm, and the lower extremities from just proximal to the toes to below the knee. The extremities appear erythematous, swollen, and scaly with multiple vesicles and areas denuded of overlying skin. The patient is insistent that the cause of her discomfort is parasites. She claims to have had this complaint constantly for 6 years, starting just after a quadruple bypass and continuing without interruption till the current visit. She reports a history of kidney failure, fatigue, and fluid retention, but denies any other symptoms.

The patient claims that her house is infested with minuscule mites that bite constantly and leave an itching welt unrelieved by any therapy. The mites appeared shortly after a quadruple bypass performed 6 years ago. Despite Mrs. Hightower having removed all furniture and carpet, and repeated exterminator attempts, the mites persist. Her husband, who brought her in today, confirms the story, and offers a sample of the mites to corroborate her story. The lesions appeared initially on her ankles bilaterally, and have spread to all four extremities. She describes the itching as constant to the point of distraction, frequently causing her to scratch till blood is drawn. The lower extremities, particularly the ankles, are red, swollen and have multiple vesicles filled with a clear fluid. The skin itself appears thickened and leathery to the touch. The edema is non-pitting, and appears more as a response to repetitive itching than an accumulation of fluid as she has maintained.

Previous physicians had prescribed anti-histamines, corticosteroids, and various antibiotics for the condition, without change in her symptoms. She states that the skin reddening and discomfort have recently grown much worse, prompting her to seek different medical attention. The inability to acquire the correct diagnosis or relief of symptoms has left the patient depressed and frustrated to the point of tears multiple times during the interview. A scraping was done for scabies along with an examination of the sample provided by the patient.

Reflections on the Case

Based on the patient's medical history, clinical picture, and absence of any mites, including the sample the husband had brought, the diagnosis of neurodermatitis was made.

Teaching Points

Neurodermatitis is a term encompassing several dermatological conditions sharing an underlying psychological basis. The disorder can result in delusions of parasitosis, lichen simplex chronicus, neurotic excoriations, or prurigo nodularis. The disorder commonly results from a cycle of idiopathic itch followed by scratching for relief of symptoms, which paradoxically worsens the itch. This cycle results in a thickening of the skin, often turning it darker and leathery. The cause of the initial itch is unknown, and often the scratch becomes a reflex rendering the initial itch inconsequential.

Various causes of the initial itch have been proposed, including irritation from fabric or insect bites, psoriasis, or atopic dermatitis. It has been particularly noted in populations of mentally retarded children with repetitive motion disorders or elderly individuals with depression or obsessive-compulsive disorder (OCD). Another hypothesis claims that it can be triggered by depression, anxiety or other psychological disorders. One of the more common manifestations of the disorder is the persistent belief that bugs are causing the itching/ lesions, and the patients frequently claim that they feel bugs crawling on them. Kidney failure, often accompanied by persistent fatigue and mild to moderate edema, can lead to multiple electrolyte disturbances, anemia, uremia, and pruritus.

This disease generally affects the elderly, and has a predilection for females. The lesions appear as hyper-pigmented, thickened skin (Fig. 10.1). There are often lesions in various states, from newly appearing erythematous macules to scars from past lesions (Fig. 10.2). They often exhibit a linear pattern, reflecting the involvement of scratching in the pathogenesis of this disorder (Fig. 10.3). The extremities are most often involved, often bilaterally (Fig. 10.4). Rarely, the genital regions may be involved.

Allergic contact dermatitis presents with many of the symptoms presented here. It is a contact dermatitis, a Type 4 hypersensitivity reaction, less commonly seen than irritant contact dermatitis. It results from two phases: the initial Induction Phase, in which the allergen is picked up by dendrites and present the allergen to T cells, and the Elicitation phase in which the previously stimulated T cells to respond by releasing large quantities of cytokines. It typically presents as a rash or lesion that itches, oozes, crusts, or develops scale. If the allergen is present chronically, the skin may even darken and thicken. Allergic contact dermatitis is distinguishable

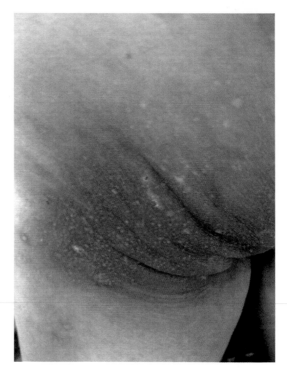

FIGURE 10.1   Neurodermatitis. Excoriated, pink papules surrounded by hyper-pigmented, thickened skin as a result of long-standing disease

from neurodermatitis by being widespread and reproducible upon exposure to the allergen. Diagnosis is commonly by history and physical exam, but a patch allergy test is often definitive.

Scabies should also be included on the list of differential diagnosis. It is a skin disorder caused by tiny mites, and the initial symptoms can mimic neurodermatitis. This mimicry can be particularly apparent when the patient presents with complaints of mites all over their house and person. Scabies affects all genders and ages, and is particularly common in nursing homes and daycares, two populations most at risk for developing neurodermatitis. Mites forming burrows in the

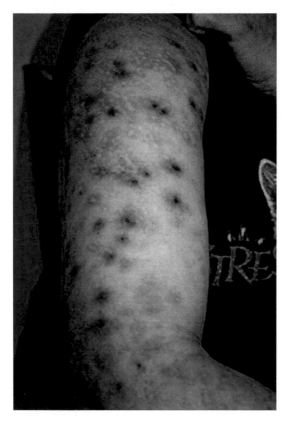

FIGURE 10.2 Neurodermatitis. Fleshly excoriated macules mixed with hyper-pigmented, post-inflammatory scars

patient's skin and then laying eggs in them are the cause of cutaneous signs and symptoms of this infestation. A portion of the damage done to the skin is from the patient scratching to relieve the itch caused by the burrows. These lesions caused by scratching can appear similar to initial lesions in neurodermatitis. Diagnosis of scabies can be accomplished by direct skin examination, microscopic examination, or biopsy.

Lichen planus is a skin disorder that presents often in patients older than 40. It affects both sexes equally, and is

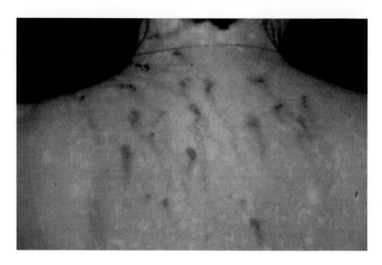

FIGURE 10.3 Neurodermatitis. Macules distributed in a linear fashion in reachable skin areas indicating scratching as part of the pathogenesis

often mistaken for other disorders. The etiology of this disorder is unknown, although genetics is thought to play a role due to familial co-occurrence. Chronic active hepatitis C is also commonly observed in these patients, leading to the theory that the virus replicates in the skin causing irritation in genetically susceptible individuals. The lesions are quite distinctive, appearing purple, popular, pruritic, polyangular, and planar. They are 2–10 mm, flat topped, purple papules covered by lacy white striae that signify epidermal thickening. Lichen planus can be diagnosed by direct biopsy.

Treatment for neurodermatitis is multifocal. Initial treatment frequently involves topical and systemic glucocorticoids, which may decrease the itching and redness of affected areas. Additionally, treatment may be aimed at decreasing depression or any psychological ailments, if present. Counseling, meditation, and relaxation training has been successful in encouraging cessation of scratching.

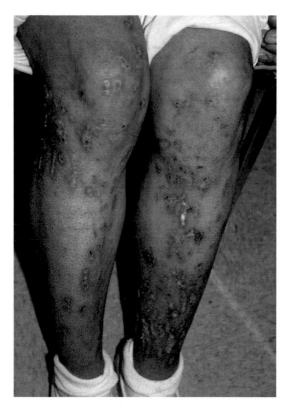

FIGURE 10.4 Neurodermatitis. Excoriated macules and papules are frequently found on the bilateral extremities

Part III
Cases of Psychocutaneous Disease

Delusions of Parasitotis: Introducing the "Spectrum of Delusional Ideation"

Articulating the Concept

The stereotype of delusional patients, such as those with delusions of parasitosis, is that they are typically utterly helpless. In reality, there is a spectrum of psychopathology ranging from formication alone to total investment in particular ideations (e.g., parasites having three antennae and five eyes) as well as in universal acceptance of these delusional thoughts (i.e., everyone has to believe the patient). This concept, herein referred to as the *"spectrum of delusional ideation"* (SDI), is of great significance because it can aid the practitioner in evaluating the patient's mindset and tailoring the therapeutic approach to his/her delusional status.

It is important to note that the psychological status of untreated patients can evolve through various stages of delusional ideation. Patients presenting with formication (i.e., crawling, biting, stinging sensations) without fixed ideas tend to be relatively manageable. Over time, they can have impairment of previously normal thought processes and become preoccupied with certain beliefs, not to mention having little tolerance for other people's opinions.

In the following six cases, we strive to first familiarize our audience with various degrees and types of delusional ideations existing within the SDI. Secondly, where possible we will make suggestions about how to successfully manage each case based on the experiences of the authors. Regrettably, patients who have been referred to our psychodermatologic clinic are frequently on the delusional end of the SDI rather than the healthier, less fixed-ideation end. So, if a patient who is somewhere in the middle of this psychopathology spectrum presents to you, please keep in mind that initiating anti-psychotic therapy as soon as possible can forestall this vicious progression toward a completely delusional state.

Interpreting Phenomenology

The specific approach to managing an SDI patient depends how delusional he/she is. If formication symptoms are the only concerns, then you can have an open discussion without having to fear offending him/her, since there are no convictions to be contradicted. On the other hand, when a patient is vexingly rigid and more ego-invested in having his/her beliefs validated than seeking symptomatic relief through trial-and-error treatment, we approach him/her differently. Even if such patient might never accept the use of medications, he/she can still be made a little more comfortable through maintenance of supportive interactions with you, as long as this task is not too taxing. If he/she is innately hostile to your attempts to connect, then you should be reconciled with the fact that he/she is beyond reach. The focus may then be shifted toward parting on an amicable basis.

The Attitude of a Practitioner

You may feel apprehensive and averse upon learning that the new patient waiting to see you is delusional. However, it is important to not let this feeling show. In many instances, patients may transfer negative feelings from previous experiences with other healthcare practitioners onto you. If this is encountered, little deeds such as greeting the patient with a welcoming demeanor, smiling warmly during the interview, or asking if the patient is comfortable can go a long way in building a good rapport with this type of patients, rather than saying "I am not Dr. So-and-so who treated you unkindly." In addition, please avoid taking the patient's rejection of your opinions as a personal affront. SDI patients tend to not be interested in what other people think – this is part of the disease process.

Even with the most sophisticated approach as outlined in this book, the authors recognize that there is a limit to how much a practitioner can do for an SDI patient and more importantly, how much patience a practitioner can have. Please understand that delusional patients have a limited capacity to recognize social norms, and may disrespect your boundaries, especially those with regards to time constraint. If you notice that a patient is making you upset, it might be in your and his/her best interests to terminate the visit and protect your sanity. For instance, if a patient is pushing you to listen to his/her narrative beyond ending time for the visit, you can politely state: "Ms. So-and-so, you have a fascinating story, and I would love to hear more about it another day. But for today, we are out of time. May I see you again in 2 weeks to continue our conversation?"

Chapter 11
Formication Without Delusions

Mr. Schmidt is a 38 year-old Caucasian man presenting with a 3-month history of extremely bothersome crawling, biting, and stinging sensations. He reported that at times he felt as if "a 1,000 bugs were falling and crawling on my [his] skin." The patient claimed that no living organisms were involved in causing his skin condition, not only because there was no evidence to suggest this but also because the symptomatology was so bizarre that he knew of no organisms likely to cause this type of discomfort. The onset of these symptoms was not correlated with any particular events or stressors, and he denied recreational drug use. Past medical history was unremarkable. Due to the intensity of the formication, he was very eager to undergo aggressive therapy to reduce these sensations.

Reflections on the Case

Formication without delusions is rarely seen in a dermatology practice. However, it is possible that many patients start out with symptoms of formication and slowly progress to developing circumscribed delusions as a way of explaining the cause of the stinging, biting, and crawling sensations. One retrospective study reported the efficacy of pimozide for what the authors referred to as the "chronic cutaneous dysesthesia syndrome," which has a symptomatology identical to formication. Seven out of seven patients treated with pimozide for this condition (excluding the patient whose main concern is photo-sensitivity) became symptom-free with follow-up periods ranging from 8 months to 5 years [22].

The authors did not disclose information related to treatment durations for these patients, nor many details regarding side effects and adverse events, save for the fact that one patient developed iatrogenic Parkinson's syndrome [22]. Out of the two psychotropic drugs that the patient was on (i.e., fluoxetine and pimozide), pimozide was most likely the culprit. Under the assumption that this was the only adverse event found in the seven patients, one can argue that pimozide is as safe as it is effective for the treatment of formication/chronic cutaneous dysesthesia syndrome.

Chapter 12
The Slightly Delusional Patient

Mrs. Wang is a 69 year-old Asian American woman presenting with a chief complaint of being "infested with parasites" for the past 5 months. She described crawling, stinging and biting sensations that occurred spontaneously all over her body. There were a few plastic zip-lock bags containing what she believes to the parasites and their eggs. From her expressions and demeanor, the patient appeared deeply worried about and quite preoccupied with her infestation. However, upon further questioning Mrs. Wang stated that she was not entirely convinced about the existence of live organisms in her skin. She was open to other explanations, but above all, just wanted to receive a good treatment.

Reflections on the Case

Considering the last statement from the above scenario, it would be difficult to know for certain whether or not Mrs. Wang is delusional. However, she brought you specimens in a plastic zip-lock bag to prove a point: the bugs are real. We refer to this as the "zip-lock bag sign;" you might also hear some practitioners say the "matchbox sign" because matchboxes

T.V. Nguyen et al., *Clinical Cases in Psychocutaneous Disease*, 55
Clinical Cases in Dermatology,
DOI 10.1007/978-1-4471-4312-3_12, © Springer-Verlag London 2014

were used before the advent of zip-lock bags. It appears that she still has some investment in the parasitic infestation theory, but on the outside she will likely concede if you challenge her belief so as to be able to receive the best care from you. This patient belongs somewhere in the middle of the SDI, probably closer to the formication-only end.

Teaching Points

Once again, we recommend medical therapy with pimozide for Mrs. Wang. She may report fewer or no symptoms after treatment with pimozide; how, it is quite likely that she will not change her mind about the having been infested with living organisms in the first place (or in the case of Morgellons Disease – with inanimate objects coming out of the skin). By official psychiatric definition, she is still delusional because she has not repudiated her fixed belief. But she no longer suffers symptoms of formication and appears uninterested in whether or not you believe her story. For all practical purposes, the treatment has been successful.

Chapter 13
The Delusional but Hopeful Patient

Ms. Alvarez, a 58 year-old Hispanic woman, presented with 2 years of "infestation with bugs." The episodes started when she stayed at her friend's house and was reportedly exposed to dirty blankets and soiled linens. She had seen many physicians, both dermatologists and non-dermatologists. She brought in a bag full of topical medications including topical steroids, anti-fungal creams, anti-bacterial ointments, and moisturizers, none of which were of benefit. She had been treated twice with permethrine (Elimite®) by a dermatologist with only transient relief of symptoms. She described in great details the life cycle and the mating habits of these parasites. She also presented to you zip-lock bags of soiled materials containing tissue papers with brown stains suspended in cloudy water. She stated unequivocally that these specimens contain the "parasites" she has described.

The patient appeared hopeful that some effective treatment might be provided. But at the same time, she also showed some hesitancy in describing the details of her condition. She stated that if she were to explain the whole phenomenon in details, then "you will probably think that I am (she is) crazy." Past medical history consisted of controlled gastroesophageal reflux disease. The patient has no previous psychiatric or substance abuse history.

Reflections on the Case

Patients with delusions of parasitosis are typically older women. In the older age group, the sex ratio is three to one with a female predominance, and the majority of the older female patients have reasonably stable social situations (i.e., being married, having good family support and stable jobs, etc.). In the experience of the authors, it is rare to see young patients present with DoP. If they do, the sex ratio in this age group is about one to one. These young patients with DoP frequently harbor problems related to substance abuse and tend to be marginally adapted to society.

Teaching Points

Once again, the "matchbox sign" or "zip-lock bag sign" is illustrated here by the fact that the patient brought in several specimens stored in such containers for you to examine. In order to establish therapeutic rapport (i.e., a trusting relationship with the patient), it is strategically critical that you actually examine them. Not looking at the specimens means that you do not believe her story, which is extremely aggravating and can aggravate Ms. Alvarez.

If she does not respect your opinions, then she will not listen to your medical advice, and thus any medication prescribed to her – even if it were the best medication available – is likely to be tossed aside. You should use the first few sessions to establish an emotional connection with the patient before putting pressure on yourself to discuss the possible institution of antipsychotic therapy. The authors hope that you will remember one important point about Ms. Alvarez' case: even though she is hopeful for symptomatic relief, she might still have a moderate degree of delusional ideation, and as a result, can be very sensitive to anything that contradicts her conviction.

Chapter 14
The *Hopelessly* Delusional Patient

Ms. Daisy is a 65 year-old Caucasian new patient, who presented with a 2-year history of being infested with "parasites." She brought with her numerous items such as impeccably prepared slides of these so-called parasite carcasses, professionally taken photographs of skin debris and other inanimate objects, and articles published in scientific journals as well as the popular press discussing parasitic infestation. She has already visited numerous dermatology practitioners and one parasitology specialist, who could not identify any ecto-parasites (i.e., those infesting visible parts of the body). Her medical history included well-controlled hypertension and chronic back pain.

During the examination, Ms. White requested that you search her skin from head to toes for evidence of living and/or dead parasites. When you offered a topical antiparasitic agent as empirical therapy (i.e., not as proof of existing parasitosis but on a trial-and-error basis), she showed no interest. In fact, all attempts at initiating her on empirical therapy were rejected, including suggestions regarding relatively benign medications such as permethrin/Crotamiton cream or lotion (Eurax®) and antipsychotic therapy for formication symptoms. You felt puzzled and a little bit frustrated. Seeing this, she tearfully

stated, "You don't understand, Doctor! I have been very
miserable for 2 years because of these bugs. I do not want
to take any drugs until I know that is living underneath
my skin. Could you please help me find them to prove
that I'm not crazy? Then we can try to get rid of them."

Reflections on the Case

For a couple of reasons, Ms. Daisy's interest in therapy pales
in comparison with her investment in conceptual validation
of her delusional parasitosis. As she is met with disbelief
those not sharing the same delusional ideation, her desire to
have such ideation validated becomes even stronger. In the
experience of the authors, cerebral patients who seem proud
of their intellectual capability frequently end up in this situation. It is very challenging for you to entice them to undergo
treatment by the possibility of symptomatic relief, simply
because the actual symptoms do not bother them as much as
not having a satisfactory explanation for such symptoms. On
the other hand, as a practitioner you should tactfully avoid
providing conceptual validation because doing so can render
their delusions even more rigid to the point of being
completely non-negotiable.

Teaching Points

The term "*hopelessly* delusional" denotes a special type of
patients at one extreme of the SDI: those who are so antago-
nistic and frequently hostile from the start that there is no
room for communication or negotiation. Luckily, these
patients are rare, and most of them are this way because their
delusional ideation were rejected or invalidated by a healthcare professional at some point during the course of their
disease. The authors believe that showing such patients a

positive attitude can help minimize the degree of "negative transference."

The word "transference" used to describe this phenomenon should not be confused with its use in a classical Freudian sense, whereby transfer of life-long feelings and perceptions is from parental figures to other authority figures. Here we refer to the transfer of feelings from the previous practitioner(s) to you. If you notice persistence of an overtly hostile attitude, the negative transference is creating problems for your relationship with the patient. As such, it is important to explicitly and diplomatically challenge the patient to reconsider her preconceived notions about you, and often the patient realizes that her negative perceptions and feelings are unwarranted. Upon such realization, some patients may even feel embarrassed.

Some patients are relatively hopeless they have already done such an extensive research on topics involving parasitosis that it is almost impossible to try to change their mind. The author (JK) has encountered rare patients who researched this topic so thoroughly that they even anticipated the author's approach (i.e., challenging and trying to modify their thinking to make it more favorable toward empirical therapy). There is not a perfect way to handle this situation, and it might be best to be honest about how you feel and find a way to part with the patient in peace, "Ms. Daisy, I am not convinced that we have uncovered the truth about your skin disease. As such, I am interested in helping you explore the true cause of your crawling, biting, and stinging sensations. In terms of what I can do to help you feel better, it is your decision to take or not to take this medication. However, I have done my best at this point. I wish there were something else I could do to improve your condition."

Chapter 15
Drug-Induced Formication and Delusions of Parasitosis

Mr. Northwood is a 25 year-old Caucasian man, who presented with a chief complaint of being infested by "bugs." He reported intense, bothersome sensations of crawling, stinging, and biting, which were felt frequently all over this body. He otherwise had a clean bill of health and denied any psychological stress or emotional issues. Upon further questioning, he admitted to regular, heavy use of cocaine for the past 2 years. After he had started experimenting with cocaine, he started to notice these symptoms, which were tolerable at the time. However, the sensations progressively worsened to the point where he could no longer resist the urge to scratch or to pick at his skin. His general practitioner could not determine the cause, and as a result, referred him to your psychodermatology clinic for help.

You gently suggested that the temporal association between his period of cocaine use and the appearance of his symptoms might explain the etiology of his condition. However, Mr. Northwood insisted that there were "bugs" involved, and brought up the fact that a few of his fellow cocaine users were noting similar symptoms suggestive of infestation. After a long discussion, you convinced him that a referral to a drug rehabilitation program was needed. As for the formication symptoms, you discussed possibly taking pimozide at the next visit, after he had had a normal electrocardiogram (EKG) test. A few weeks later, you were notified that Mr. Northwood never showed up to his initial visit at the rehab facility. Thereafter, all attempts to reach the patient were not successful.

Reflections on the Case

Formication has been associated with the use of certain recreational drugs, such as cocaine, amphetamine, and narcotics. Patients who are dependent on alcohol tend to experience visual DoP not during periods of alcohol use but during periods of alcohol withdrawal. Of note, a number of medical conditions can also cause the DoP-type clinical picture, including but not limited to B12 or folate deficiency, thyroid abnormality, etc.

"Cocaine bug" is a commonly used term among cocaine users who frequently experience formication from cocaine use. Fortunately, most of these cocaine users know that the formication is from cocaine and not from a real-life situation. In rare instances that are typically seen with chronic drug abuse, a small portion of cocaine users may develop full-blown delusional parasitosis and come to believe that they are truly infested [23]. This has been reported in a couple experiencing a shared delusion associated with cocaine use [24]. The case described above was chosen deliberately for Mr. Northwood's imperfect insight because those with clear insight regarding the drug-induced nature of their symptoms are unlikely to seek help from a dermatologic practitioner.

It is important to be mindful about Mr. Northwood's sensitivity surrounding his history of multi-recreational drug use. If you phrase your questions as blunt and forceful requests, he may become defensive and deny any drug use altogether.

It may be wise to ask questions about his recreational drug use very nonchalantly – as if this is simply an effort on your part to obtain information about every patient's medical history in a thorough fashion. He may find it comfortably acceptable if questions about his recreational drug use are conducted in a mechanical fashion, following routine questions about his general health (i.e., sleep, appetite, etc.) as well as any history of over-the-counter and prescription drug use.

In terms of management, the first and the foremost intervention is to get these patients to discontinue the current drug abuse. Without detoxification, there is no reliable solution to their condition. Moreover, chronic drug users commonly abuse multiple recreational substances, as illustrated by the case of Mr. Northwood, who admitted to using narcotics in addition to cocaine. This renders the use of pimozide risky even for symptomatic relief, since pimozide is known to have opiate blocking effects and can precipitate withdrawal reactions depending on the degree to which the patient is addicted to the narcotics.

It is an unfortunate fact that drug abusers, similar to alcoholics, are typically resistant to accepting help. Nevertheless, referrals to detoxification programs should still be made with much enthusiasm and encouragement on your part. Even though these patients may not follow up with your referrals within a reasonable time frame, with enough accumulated difficulty in life, they will eventually commit to receiving professional help. A useful analogy that the author (JK) frequently employs is that of a stonecutter, who may strike a large stone many times at first with no visible effects. After numerous strikes, the stone suddenly splits open. This is to say that the practitioner should not feel discouraged about the initial resistance from the recalcitrant drug-abusing patient.

Chapter 16
Other Delusionoid Beliefs

Mrs. Aaron is a 56 year-old African-American woman, who presented with a chief complaint of a constant sensation of being covered by "cobwebs" on her face for the past 8 months. She did not seen any spiders or insects nearby when this sensation occurred, and appeared unconcerned about the possibility of an infestation. Upon examination, she showed no primary skin lesions but was observed to wipe her face with her hand frequently as if to get rid of these cobwebs. She related that due to the intensity of the cobweb sensation, she had not been able to focus on any task – which had hindered her from gaining employment since the start of her disease.

At the end of the visit, Mrs. Aaron agreed to undergo treatment with pimozide at a low starting dose of 1 mg/day. The dosage was increased by an increment of 1 mg/month to 3 mg/day, and she stayed on this dose for 3 months. Her symptom had decreased significantly upon reaching the 3 mg/day dose and had disappeared completely after the 3-month period. Seeing that she had recovered from her disease, you decided to taper off the pimozide dosage while monitoring aggressively for recurrence (fortunately, none was found). According to the latest follow-up record, she remained symptom-free 1 year after finishing therapy, had begun a new job, and described her life as being "very enjoyable."

Reflections on the Case

DoP is the most common manifestation of a category of disorders classified in Europe as monosymptomatic hypochondriacal psychosis (MHP). The authors have seen many variations of MHP, including patients who are convinced that they are losing hair (when they are actually not), those believing that their skin is too greasy (when it is not), etc. Fortunately, pimozide and possibly other anti-psychotic agents appear to be quite effective for a wide spectrum of MHP manifestations, reaching beyond the classic symptomatology of parasitosis. This is because such medications may have very broad anti-psychotic effects.

Sensing cobwebs, perceiving hair loss, and excessive greasiness when there is none are examples of self-perception disturbances. In other words, there appears to be a disconnect between what actually exists in reality and the information produced by the brain after aberrant processing of such reality. This can be likened to a "vintage" television set made a few decades ago that produces double images when broken. The quick and easy fix was achieved by knocking on the television set until the double image disappeared. In an analogous manner, anti-psychotic agents such as pimozide perform a similar function of resetting the connection between the outer reality and a patient's inner representation of it. The proper approach to convince Mrs. Aaron to try pimozide can be likened to that prescribed in the above cases of DoP, depending on the degree of her conviction in the delusion.

Neurotic Excoriations

A Misnomer?

The authors have some concerns regarding whether or not the terminology "neurotic excoriations" is a misnomer, since not all triggers for excoriating behavior are neurotic in origin. In fact, there are several possible underlying psychiatric processes causing patients to excoriate, including but not limited to emotional stress, anxiety, and underlying major depressive episodes. Intense focal cutaneous dysesthesia as described in the above case is also a common cause for neurotic excoriations. Rarely, patients with psychotic ideation excoriate typically due to the belief that they have to remove something from the skin in order for it to heal or function normally.

The term "neurotic excoriations" lumps all of the aforementioned underlying processes into one category of neurosis, which is not only an inadequate but also an incorrect explanation. Therefore, it is important to take the diagnostic label "neurotic excoriations" with a grain of salt and dig deeper into the patient's narrative. Sadly, we often hear from patients that their practitioners have failed to ask simple, important questions that could have revealed the triggers for their excoriating behavior, and instead assumed that the self-induced damage to their skin could only be caused by psychosis. Some of these patients have even been given unfortunate labels, such as "psychotic" and "crazy." We encourage you to openly, explicitly, and thoroughly investigate the cause for your patient's excoriating behavior without any presumed notions.

Chapter 17
Neurotic Excoriations Secondary to Cutaneous Dysesthesia

Ms. Ellington is 34 year-old Caucasian woman presenting with a 1-year history of excoriations on easily reachable areas of the face, neck, dorsal hands, lateral arms, and upper chest. She had been referred to the psychodermatology clinic with an initial diagnosis of "psychosis." There were no primary skin lesions as noted on the previous physical exam in her records. During the interview, she clearly appeared both embarrassed and apologetic about picking at her skin. She showed no elaborate ideation regarding the reason for her behavior. However, after you asked, "can you tell me exactly what makes you pick your skin?" She reports an intense focal pain in her skin as the cause.

The patient described the pain as "if somebody is sticking me [her] with a needle," or "like getting an electric shock repeatedly in the same place on my [her] skin." From the onset of her condition, the intense focal pain had been the main trigger. She discovered that by excoriating the skin she was able to ameliorate or temporarily eliminate the pain. All attempts to use topical medications, both prescription and over the counter, have failed to adequately control it. Although the patient felt awful about the extent of self-induced damage to her skin, she could not think of any other way to get relief.

Gleaning from Ms. Ellington's past medical records, various diagnoses were given, including "psychosis," "delusional disorder," "neurotic excoriations," and "lichen simplex chronicus/neurodermatitis." Interestingly, none of the previous practitioners noted cutaneous pain as the primary trigger of her condition.

Teaching Points

As stated earlier, cutaneous dysesthesia is not an uncommon reason for excoriation. If this is the case, it is important to first obtain a neurology consult, since many neurological conditions ranging from peripheral neuropathy to early manifestations of multiple sclerosis can present as cutaneous dysesthesia. Moreover, a third of the cases of multiple sclerosis initially present with only cutaneous dysesthesia frequently not following dermatomal patterns. Even psychiatrists at times make the mistake of diagnosing early multiple sclerosis as psychiatric disorders.

If a neurologist feels confident that the underlying pathology is a neurological condition, then he or she should manage the case. However, this is rare. Frequently, the author (JK) has observed that the neurologist loses interest in such as case as Ms. Ellington's and discharges the patient without any diagnosis or therapeutic suggestions. It may be helpful to treat her symptoms empirically with gabapentin or a tricyclic anti-depressant (e.g., amitryptilline, despiramine, etc.) at a low dose of 10–15 mg/day for the analgesic effect. If neither gabapentin nor tricyclic anti-depressants (TCAs) prove to be efficacious, then an SSRI can be tried with the understanding that the analgesic effect of SSRIs is not as well substantiated for cutaneous dysesthesia as that of gabapentin or TCAs.

Chapter 18
Neurotic Excoriations Secondary to Underlying Major Depression

Mr. Adams is 27 year-old Caucasian new patient, who presented to the dermatology clinic with several excoriations on the face, arms, and legs. The lesions were all located on easily reachable areas of his anatomy such as the extensor arms but not the medial arms, the anterior legs but not the posterior legs, etc. No primary skin lesions were seen. The patient was visibly depressed. However, when asked what was causing him to be distressed, he answered: "nothing other than having these spots on my [his] skin." The practitioner, sensing that forward questions might not be useful, decided to change the questioning approach and asked about his general wellbeing. The patient then reported severe early insomnia (i.e., he cannot fall asleep), middle insomnia (i.e., he wakes up frequently in the middle of the night), and terminal insomnia (i.e., he wakes up early in the morning and cannot go back to sleep even despite being extremely tired).

Next, the patient was asked, "what is going on in your life?" to which he responded, "Doctor, I'm in an abusive relationship. And these spots on my skin – they started to appear after my girlfriend and I began fighting." By this time, the patient was tearful and no longer denied

T.V. Nguyen et al., *Clinical Cases in Psychocutaneous Disease*, 73
Clinical Cases in Dermatology,
DOI 10.1007/978-1-4471-4312-3_18, © Springer-Verlag London 2014

that there was nothing wrong in his life. He was started on doxepin at 10 mg at bedtime, and the dose was gradually titrated up by 10–20 mg every 3 weeks to the anti-depressant dose of 100 mg per day. During the titration period, his sleep pattern, anxiety and agitation dramatically improved. Approximately a month after the anti-depressant dose was reached, the patient recovered from depression, and his excoriating behavior stopped completely.

Reflections on the Case

It is not uncommon for underlying depression to be associated with excoriation. The diagnostic term "depressive excoriation" has been proposed by one of the authors (JK) to distinguish it from neurotic excoriations and to highlight the importance of depression as the underlying cause of this particular subtype of excoriation. Depressed patients sometimes report cutaneous dysesthesia of a very painful and focal nature as in the previous case; however, excoriation secondary to depression is not necessarily associated with cutaneous dysesthesia. As illustrated in the above case, these patients frequently deny psychological distress as the primary underlying trigger for their excoriating behavior. Many actually prefer to think that the excoriation is responsible for their emotional turmoil.

In psychiatry, the term "somatization" refers to the phenomenon, where patients are thought to be using a physical complaint as a screen to hide a serious, intractable psychological issue that they would consciously or unconsciously rather not deal with. In a somewhat twisted way, this defense mechanism can be adaptive since such distorted perception in the patient's mind protects him from feeling the full blunt of his issues. Ironically, the defense mechanism if frequently viewed as maladaptive from the practitioner's point of view, since it hinders disclosure of the truth to establish therapeutic rapport.

Teaching Points

For the aforementioned reasons, if you can represent a supportive, reliable, and non-judgmental figure in his life, Mr. Adams may become willing to forgo his defense mechanism and tell the truth. If this occurs, you must be ready to accept his psychological revelation and allow for frequent follow-ups to provide emotional support. If the patient is in need of additional psychological counseling, it is appropriate to refer him to a mental health professional with his permission.

Assessing for insomnia can be a useful strategy to corroborate the working diagnosis of underlying major depression. Of the three different types of insomnia, terminal insomnia, in which the patient wakes up early in the morning and cannot return to sleep despite being very tired, is most indicative of underlying depression. Doxepin, a TCA with a potent sedative property, is used for its quadruple therapeutic effects (i.e., anti-depressant, anti-anxiety/agitation, anti-histamine/anti-pruritic, and hypnotic). Even though the anti-depressant effect generally does not become evident until the patient has been on a dose of 100 mg/day or more for several weeks, the other effects can be observed at lower doses. For any patient with major depression, it is critical to ascertain and clearly document that the patient does not have suicidal ideation. In fact, it is well justified to follow him up once weekly to ensure that he receives frequently emotional support and to avoid dispensing a large supply of doxepin at once.

When patients are truly and deeply depressed, they can appear indifferent to the pain associated with their excoriating behavior. They may make facial expressions indicating pain while excoriating their skin but will deny any associated pain or discomfort. Rarely and remarkably, the authors have observed the extreme cases, where patients excoriated their skin down to the bone without being concerned about pain. It has been speculated that the release of endogenous endorphins in times of stress blunts the perception of cutaneous pain. Once the major depression has improved, skin-picking behavior stops for two reasons: first, the psychological distress is no longer manifesting as a somatic issue, and second, the patient is no longer protected from perceiving the pain in his skin.

Chapter 19
Neurotic Excoriations with Underlying Psychosis

Mr. Tran is a 72 year-old Asian American man presenting with numerous excoriations limited to the extensor
aspects of the forearms. Upon questioning, the patient
stated that there were "slivers" of foreign materials
imbedded in his skin, and he insists that they must be
taken out, or else "my [his] skin will not work normally."
His mental preoccupation with said slivers had been
going on for about 3 years, corroborated by chronic scars
running down both of his forearms. Past medical history
was remarkable for controlled hypertension and dyslip-
idemia, with no previous psychiatric history.

X-ray evaluation and skin biopsies showed no foreign materials. However, the patient dismissed these
negative results, claiming that the slivers could not be
visualized using X-rays and "are too deep to reach with
the skin biopsy probes." After much convincing on your
part, he agreed to undergo empirical treatment with
pimozide. Pimozide dosage was gradually titrated from
a 1 mg/day to 3 mg/day; as a result, he experienced
noticeable symptomatic relief. The patient happily
reported spending less time trying to remove the foreign objects from his skin and more time on leisurely
activities compared with before starting pimozide, and

T.V. Nguyen et al., *Clinical Cases in Psychocutaneous Disease*, 77
Clinical Cases in Dermatology,
DOI 10.1007/978-1-4471-4312-3_19, © Springer-Verlag London 2014

he incurred no extrapyramidal side effects during the trial period. After several months of taking pimozide at the 3 mg/day dose, he was slowly taken off the medication because his mental preoccupation and excoriating behavior had stopped.

Reflections on the Case

As this and the previous two cases illustrate, there are many possible underlying psychiatric processes responsible for neurotic excoriations, including but not limited to cutaneous dysesthesia, depression, and psychosis. Therefore, it is crucial to exhaustively inquire into the cause of each patient's excoriating behavior, since elucidating the nature of the underlying psychopathology can help you determine the most appropriate therapeutic approach. For instance, if the patient is mainly affected by cutaneous dysesthesia, then the preferred approach should involve a complete neurological evaluation and treatment with analgesics. On the other hand, if the underlying psychopathology is depression, then the first line medication to reduce depressive symptoms as well as abolish the excoriation is likely to be an anti-depressant.

Teaching Points

Mr. Tran's case represents a common scenario encountered by the authors. If a practitioner were to simply make a diagnosis based on the patient's skin findings alone, then the diagnosis could well be "neurotic excoriations." But because he also presents with a fixed delusion, a diagnosis of MHP or Morgellons Disease can also be considered. Of note, Morgellons Disease is not an officially sanctioned diagnostic term but has been commonly used by both patients and many practitioners to refer to the phenomenon, in which "fibers" allegedly extrude from the skin. Pimozide or another anti-psychotic agent (e.g., risperidone) is a logical choice as the first line treatment. When such a medication manifests its therapeutic effects, the patient typically exhibits gradual decrease in mental preoccupation about the concern, becomes less agitated, and is more able to focus on other activities. However, as stated earlier in the DoP section, he may never change his mind about the validity of the original delusional ideation.

Cutaneous Manifestations of Obsessive-Compulsive Disorder

Patients with OCD generally have more insight about their conditions than those suffering from personality disorders, depressive disorders or psychosis, etc. As a dermatology practitioner, you may encounter various skin manifestations of obsessive-compulsive spectrum disorder, ranging from acne excoriée, trichotillomania (hair pulling), onychophagia (excessive nail biting/eating) and onychotillomania (pulling of nails) to factitial dermatitis. Therapeutic options for such conditions are also varied, including mental state optimization, non-pharmacologic therapy (e.g., behavior modification therapy), pharmacotherapy, or a combination of the afore-listed approaches.

Generally, insight-oriented counseling may be the most critical step toward correcting this type of psychodermatologic disorder. Some patients require more in terms of therapy, such as a combination of non-pharmacologic and pharmacotherapy, to eliminate the compulsive behavior. If patients with OCD affecting the skin come to you for help, they most likely are aware of the need to stop the obsessive thoughts/compulsive behavior and might have made some effort on their own toward this goal. Insight-oriented therapy will not be as big of an issue for these patients as it is for those lacking in motivation, such as teenagers dragged into the office by their parents for help with their acne excoriée or trichotillomania. It may be wise to establish rapport with motivation-lacking patients on a one-on-one basis, so please do not be afraid to ask the guardians or any other parties to step outside the room during the medical interview.

One caveat to keep in mind: while patients might seek help from you regarding the cutaneous manifestations of their disease, they can be totally unaware of their non-skin-related OCD behaviors, including commonly encountered ones such as excessive hand-washing or collecting/hoarding habits. Such cases require the help of a mental health professional, such as a psychiatry practitioner, to target the pathology that runs deep beneath the surface. Another common thing to be aware of is that patients with OCD tend to begin forming compulsive behavior at a young age, and sometimes as an outlet for psychosocial disturbances (e.g., being bullied, self image issues, parents' marital conflicts, etc.). Considering the global context of their OCD behaviors, please ask the patients and their families for permission to involve other types of mental health consultants. This can optimize the therapeutic outcome of whatever you are able to provide them.

In the following cases, we hope to illustrate common scenarios of the obsessive-compulsive spectrum disorder manifesting as dermatoses, as well as offer concrete examples of therapeutic approaches to eliminate compulsive behaviors involving the skin.

Chapter 20
Acne Excoriée

Ms. Phillips is a 23-year-old Caucasian female, who presented with worsening facial acne despite being on topical and oral anti-acne medications for the past 6 months. The papules presented mostly on her forehead, cheeks, and chins, and seemed to be multiplying rapidly. Many of such papules appeared red and filled with yellow pus in the center, whereas others were forming "ugly" scars as they healed. The patient stated that she could not help thinking about the papules after seeing them in the mirror. She was not sure how frequently she acted on the impulses to touch them. According to her mother, the face touching occurred all day long.

Patient had a clean bill of health otherwise. She claimed that work at the car dealership had been stressful, as her boss had been pushing her and other employees to stay late in order to make more car sales. She continued to search for a suitable mental health professional but had yet to find one. When asked how long this increase in stress at work had been going on, the patient responded, "oh, maybe 6, 7 months. These last two quarters have been unbearable."

T.V. Nguyen et al., *Clinical Cases in Psychocutaneous Disease*, 81
Clinical Cases in Dermatology,
DOI 10.1007/978-1-4471-4312-3_20, © Springer-Verlag London 2014

Reflections on the Case

A patient with acne excoriée most commonly presents as a young Caucasian female with excoriated acne and scars. As a result of the self-inflicting nature of the condition, patients will tend to excoriate regions that are more easily accessible. Therefore, the distribution of scars or excoriations over the body can provide a useful clue to clinicians. The patient with acne excoriée can have a distribution of lesions resembling the shape of butterfly wings on the back, referred to as the "butterfly sign." In the butterfly sign, there is sparing of the upper, lateral sides of the back bilaterally resulting from the fact that the patient cannot reach these areas. Similarly, there tends to be more involvement of the extensor arm as compared to the medial arm, and more involvement of the anterior thigh as compared to the posterior thigh. Often, patients report a sense of tension immediately prior to picking at their skin, and a sense of relief after the behavior is complete [25].

Teaching Points

Acne excoriée is a psychodermatological condition that refers to the behavior of picking acne lesions. The primary pathophysiologic source is in the psyche and not in the skin. Acne excoriée is characterized by picking or scratching at acne or skin with minor epidermal abnormalities [26]. It is an acne-involved subtype of excoriating behavior referred to by various names such as neurotic excoriation, psychogenic excoriation, pathological/compulsive skin picking, or dermatotillomania.

Though the patient has a skin condition, there is a primary psychiatric disturbance focusing on acne. The disturbance can simply be the habit of picking; however, there can also be a more serious source for the behavior. Patients with acne excoriée can have a variety of underlying psychopathology, but depression and anxiety appear to be the two most common underlying psychiatric conditions. Many patients also report compulsion for picking at the skin associated with poor self-image [27]. The formation of scars as a result of excoriation causes even more negative psychosocial impact, further exacerbating social isolation, depression, and anxiety, thereby leading to a vicious cycle.

Approximately 2 % of dermatology clinic patients are found to have some form of psychogenic excoriation [26]. The age of onset of the condition typically ranges from 15 to 45 years, and the duration of symptoms has a range of 5 and 21 years [26]. Though onset of this condition generally occurs in adulthood, acne excoriée is one of the most common presentations of psychodermatology in the pediatric age group [27]. There is an increase in females compared to males with acne excoriée, and the female to male ratio for all psychogenic excoriations is 8:1 [25, 26]. There are more case studies in the literature involving Caucasian patients with acne excoriée compared with African Americans or other racial groups, but there are no confirmatory studies of racial distribution in the general population. In addition, the lifetime prevalence of the condition is unknown.

Patients with acne excoriée can have comorbidity of mood and anxiety disorders, and thus present with severe psychosocial impairment. Mood disorders are found in 48–68 % of patients and include major depression, dysthymia (persistent mild depression), and bipolar disorders [28, 29]. Anxiety disorders are found in 41–65 % of patients, and include generalized anxiety disorder, agoraphobia, panic disorder, social and more specific phobia, obsessive-compulsive disorder, and post-traumatic stress disorder [29, 30]. Additionally, if a patient has a mood or anxiety disorder, he or she frequently has other psychiatric disorders related to the mood or anxiety disorder, particularly a compulsive-impulsive spectrum disorder, including body dysmorphic disorder, eating disorder, substance use disorder, or an impulse control disorder, which includes kleptomania, compulsive buying, and trichotillomania [31]. For very rare patients, acne excoriée may even present as a manifestation of a delusional disorder [32].

Significant functional impairment is a common occurrence. Patients are often embarrassed to admit their behavior to a physician. Many report impairment in social functioning including avoidance of activities that expose their skin to the public, such as sexual activity, going to the beach, and attending sports and community events [26, 33]. Patients will often use cosmetics, bandages, and clothing to hide their excoriations.

As a result of the psychiatric nature of the condition, there are no laboratory measures to make the diagnosis of acne excoriée. Instead, diagnosis is based on clinical presentation. The approach that we recommend includes taking a thorough history, conducting a detailed physical examination, and assessing the patient for an underlying psychiatric disorder that may be related to the condition. In particular, evaluating the patient for the exact nature of the underlying psychopathology such as depression, anxiety, and OCD is key.

In order to evaluate the patient for major depression or depression-related disorder, ask the patient about subjective and physiological symptoms of depression. Subjective symptoms include but are not restricted to depressed mood, excessive guilt, anhedonia, worthlessness, hopelessness, helplessness, and crying spells. Physiological symptoms of depression share such features as loss of appetite, hyperphagia, insomnia, hypersomnia, fatigue, memory loss, poor concentration, and psychomotor agitation or retardation. In order to assess the patient for anxiety, ask the patient about feeling tense or restless, becoming easily fatigued, difficulty concentrating, irritability, significant muscle tension, and difficulty sleeping. In order to evaluate the patient for OCD, inquire about repugnant thoughts and compulsive behaviors. OCD patients can be distinguished from delusional patients by retention of insight that their behavior is destructive. OCD patients believe that their behavior is damaging, in contrast to delusional patients, who have no insight and believe that what they are doing to the skin is justified no matter how destructive the behavior.

Due to the nature of the disorder, therapy targeting the psyche can help decrease destructive behavior involved in acne excoriée. For a patient with depression as the underlying cause of the acne excoriée, an anti-depressant with psychotherapy can be provided [34, 35]. A patient with anxiety as the underlying source for acne excoriée can use an anti-anxiolytic medication combined with psychotherapy. Patients with obsessive thoughts and compulsive urges to damage the skin may find relief through an anti-OCD medication such as paroxetine (Paxil®) and fluoxetine (Prozac®) along with behavioral therapy to reduce the obsessions and compulsions [26, 36]. Behavioral therapy is generally thought to be more efficacious for the treatment of OCD than insight-oriented psychotherapy [37]. For mixed depression-OCD patients, SSRIs are the preferred choice of therapy because of their dual anti-depressant and anti-OCD properties [32]. In general, SSRIs are commonly used to treat patients in dermatology with psychiatric co-morbidity, especially major depressive disorder [33, 34]. It is important to understand that pharmacologic therapy alone may not be effective if the patient is not motivated to control the compulsive urges such as a case in which a teenager is brought in by his parents. If the clinician perceives a "power struggle" between the teenager and the parent over the issue of excoriation, it is often helpful to see the teenager alone and first try to build therapeutic rapport with the teenage patient. This may help the dermatology practitioner avoid being seen and treated as another "authority figure" by the teenage patient.

Case reports have also documented efficacy of pulsed dye laser irradiation along with cognitive psychotherapy. Treatment of hypertrophic scars and acne lesions with laser was first introduced with argon laser [38]. In a case series, 585-nm flashlamp-pumped pulsed dye with concomitant cognitive psychodynamic therapy were used to stop skin picking and scar formation in two OCD patients with acne excoriée [39]. In the cases, practical behavior modification techniques, including removal of mirrors in the home and avoidance of situations that would induce stress or conflict, were helpful.

Finally, biofeedback techniques and hypnosis have also been documented to improve acne excoriée and other dermatoses with a psychological component [40]. Post-hypnotic suggestion has also been used to treat the condition. In two case reports, patients were instructed to remember the word "scar" when they felt the urge to pick at the face and to state "scar" as a reminder to refrain from picking. In both cases, acne excoriée resolved [40]. Aversion therapy techniques and habit reversal have been noted in case reports as successful strategies for cognitive-behavioral therapy [41–43]. Aversion therapy occurs when self-destructive behavior is linked to an aversive stimulus. Habit reversal treatment involves making the patient aware of the scratching behavior, teaching the patient about the negative social impact of the habit, and developing competing response of isometric exercise using fist clenching to prevent scratching.

It is important to understand the clinical presentation and work-up of a patient with acne excoriée as the underlying source of the condition can be found in the psychopathology. Working closely with the patient to serve his or her specific needs and establishing a solid therapeutic alliance can significantly improve outcomes with all treatments.

Chapter 21
Trichotillomania

Tracy is a well-appearing 16 year-old African American girl, who was brought to the dermatology clinic by her parents for gradual hair loss on the scalp. Physical exam revealed three asymmetric, incompletely hairless patches with irregular borders near the anterior hairline, to the right of the vertex, and near the left posterior hairline. The random distribution was bizarre enough to raise suspicion for self-induced alopecia. During the interview, the parents of the teenage girl were doing all of the talking with her staying quiet and wearing a countenance of resentment. When you asked her directly about possible hair-pulling behavior, she responded with a curt "no" and refused to elaborate further on her response. At one point she explicitly stated that she resented her parents for making her come to this visit. Her past medical history was otherwise unremarkable.

Next, you politely asked the parents to leave the room and wait outside. During this short period of more personal, private interaction, she revealed to the practitioner that she had indeed been pulling her hair. As such, a diagnosis of trichotillomania was made. Tracy agreed to follow up with you regularly and individually. Once the parents were brought back into the room, you earnestly explained

T.V. Nguyen et al., *Clinical Cases in Psychocutaneous Disease*,   87
Clinical Cases in Dermatology,
DOI 10.1007/978-1-4471-4312-3_21, © Springer-Verlag London 2014

to them the need to see the patient one on one during future visits, and they cheerfully accepted such suggestion. Throughout a series of subsequent visits, she changed from being suspicious and reticent with you at first to ultimately volunteering information about her hair-pulling behavior and other aspects of her personal life.

Meanwhile, you found it helpful to state explicitly and repeatedly that you had no intention to represent yet another "authority figure" in her life. Her history of illness became more complete and accurate, including the fact that the hair pulling started after a member of the opposite sex had rejected her. She also related other emotional challenges of being a teenager, such as her sense of insecurity regarding self-esteem and personal identity. It also became apparent that much of the abnormal behavior occurred automatically; therefore, she was not aware of the total duration of her hair-pulling episodes.

In terms of intervention for her trichotillomania, Tracy agreed to undergo psychotherapy with a mental health professional, and the appropriate referral was made. In addition, you recommended her to wear a digital watch that could chime on the hour to remind her not to pull her hair. Gradually, she noted that her hands were not near her scalp. For the instances where she was subconsciously engaged in the behavior as the watch chimed, the patient stopped pulling her hair, took out a pen and wrote in a small pocket notebook the possible trigger for that episode.

The trigger turned out to be of various nature, including boredom, intra-psychic stressors (i.e., thinking about something unpleasant), or extra-psychic (i.e., real-life) stressors. Even when she could not think of any obvious trigger, the very fact that she was alerted by her watch to notate the possible proximate cause appeared to help diminish the behavior. Eventually, with both ongoing psychotherapy and increased awareness, trichotillomania was brought under control, and she re-grew her hair. More importantly, the patient appeared happier and better adjusted than before.

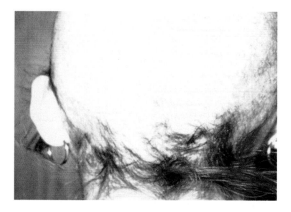

FIGURE 21.1 Trichotillomania. Partial alopecia as a result of pathologic hair pulling

Reflections on the Case

Even though many patients with trichotillomania (Fig. 21.1) readily admit to the self-inflicted nature of the condition, there are instances where the practitioner is faced with a flat denial. Such denial is even more difficult to overcome in the context of a power struggle between a teenager and her parents. In such a situation as described above, the most critical factor is whether you can establish therapeutic rapport individually with the patient, and this might mean asking the parents to leave the interview room. It is also helpful for you to explicitly and proactively communicate to her that you are not at all interested in being another authority figure dictating what she must do. Of course, such communication needs to be sincere.

Once the therapeutic rapport is established, then you can find out what exactly has been going on with this patient. If the underlying psychopathology proves to be depression or an OCD spectrum disorder, the use of anti-depressants or anti-OCD medications may be indicated. However, as in the above case, her trichotillomania is a result of real-world interpersonal and developmental difficulties; thus, referral for counseling or psychotherapy is indicated. In general, counseling and psychotherapy are more appropriate when there is a clearly defined issue needing discussion, whereas pharmacologic therapies are more appropriate when the source of the psychopathology appears to be endogenous. Of note, medications can also be effective for conditions induced by situational difficulties.

Frequently, patients engage in hair-pulling behavior automatically and almost unconsciously, especially in longstanding cases. It is very difficult to modify automatic and unconscious behavior without increasing patient awareness. Toward this end, using a digital watch that chimes on the hour is one of many creative strategies to help remind the patient about her hair-pulling behavior. In rare cases, the authors have observed that this strategy alone proves sufficient to result in complete extinction of such behavior. Unfortunately, the majority of patients still require interventions beyond increasing awareness, such as non-pharmacologic therapy or pharmacotherapy.

In terms of non-pharmacologic therapy, we want to highlight one technique involving behavior modification. You can help the patient direct attention to the obsessive thoughts and learn to re-gain control over the compulsive behaviors stemming from such thoughts using the "5-min rule." First, ask patients to pay attention to obsessive thoughts occurring throughout the day as much as possible. Once they develop awareness of these thoughts, ask them to place a 5-min interval between the thoughts and the actions that follow. The goal is to execute this practice until the patients can abstain from the compulsive behaviors, so in the beginning it may be reasonable to expect them to still carry out the actions after the waiting interval. Additionally, if 5 min prove to be too long of a waiting time for a very strong impulse, you can modify the interval to three or even 1 min to start with. As the patients perfect the exercise, you can move up the time interval ladder, adding more minutes until they can no longer keep track of time until the compulsive behaviors occur. Frequently, this means they are learning to not act on their impulses.

Chapter 22
Body Dysmorphic Disorder

Ms. Rose is a 36 year-old attractive Caucasian woman, who presented with "numerous sun spots" appearing within the last 2 years on the face. She reported that these sunspots had been increasing in number and causing her significant psychological distress, as she felt compelled to check on them constantly (i.e., spending hours in the bathroom inspecting these spots). She had no other medical problems. She was not on any medications and denied any recreational drug use. Physical examination revealed nearly perfect skin with no grossly visible lesions. Yet, she reported having seen several dermatologists and plastic surgeons because she felt depressed about her sunspots.

Even though delusional ideation was a possible diagnosis, none of the above practitioners confronted Ms. Rose directly with the fact that her skin was clear. She was started on paroxetine (Paxil®) at 20 mg/day for several months with neither side effects nor benefits. In view of the fact that she was still depressed and preoccupied with the compulsion to check her skin, you decided to increase the dose of her paroxetine by 10 mg every 3 weeks. Eventually, the maximal U.S. Food and Drug Administration (FDA)-approved dosage of

60 mg per day for OCD was reached, and after several weeks of being on this dose, the patient showed much improvement with regard to both her depression and her compulsion. As such, she has been more able to function at work and to enjoy life.

Reflections on the Case

Body dysmorphic disorder (BDD), similar to delusions of parasitosis, is a spectrum composed of different degrees of mental preoccupation, ranging from slightly abnormal perception to complete delusion regarding body dysmorphia. In fact, if the patient is completely delusional, a more specific terminology is "delusion of dysmorphosis." The challenge is to distinguish between extreme OCD from delusional disorder. This distinction cannot always be made. However, a totally delusional patient tends to have a more elaborate ideation and shows no hint of apology or embarrassment, whereas a patient with extreme OCD might demonstrate partially preserved insight.

Teaching Points

Ms. Rose did not have elaborate ideation beyond her perception of sun spots, and she did show some insight into her psychological condition. Therefore, the authors recommend giving her the diagnosis of obsessive-compulsive disorder rather than delusion of dysmorphosis. The first choice of intervention is to gradually increase her paroxetine dose rather than to add another agent such as an anti-psychotic. Even though the maximal FDA-indicated dosage of paroxetine for depression is 50 mg/day and that for OCD is 60 mg/day, the dosages used by some practitioners to improve OCD spectrum disorders can sometimes be too low to be therapeutic. This is perhaps due to the misunderstanding that the same anti-depressant dose will have the same effect for OCD;

however, it is a well-known fact in psychiatry that the dosages of anti-depressants used to treat OCD tend to be much higher than the dosages of the same agents used to treat depression. As our case illustrates, Ms. Rose had only been given 20 mg/day of paroxetine; therefore, we simply titrated up the dosage to achieve its therapeutic effects.

Once the patient is neither obsessed with her sunspots nor feels the compelled to constantly check her skin, the problem is solved! This does not mean that she will automatically reverse the belief that these lesions actually existed in the first place. For practical purposes, whether or not she believes in their existence becomes irrelevant to you. As such, the authors advise against confronting and challenging her with the fact that her skin has always been clear. Doing this might jeopardize your future therapeutic rapport with Ms. Rose.

Chapter 23
Factitial Dermatitis

Conor is an 18 year-old Caucasian man presenting with bizarrely shaped skin ulcerations on his forearms and anterior legs bilaterally. His skin lesions exhibited sharp angulations and straight edges, and some lesions had healed over with scarring, suggesting the chronicity of the condition. He had no other medical problems and was not on any medications. Upon questioning, he initially related a very vague, illogical story about the origin of the skin lesions. He neither denied nor confirmed the possible self-induced element involved.

Of note, a psychiatrist had evaluated Conor a few years prior to coming to see you, and at that point the possible diagnosis of schizotypal personality was proposed. The patient reported being very interested in magic and subject matters dealing with supernatural phenomena, having very few friends, living at home with his parents, and not having been productively employed for several years. Symptomatic care such as topical and oral antibiotics to prevent infection of his ulcerations has been provided. Most importantly, you have shown a non-judgmental, supportive stance toward his skin condition at each visit.

T.V. Nguyen et al., *Clinical Cases in Psychocutaneous Disease*,   95
Clinical Cases in Dermatology,
DOI 10.1007/978-1-4471-4312-3_23, © Springer-Verlag London 2014

After several such supportive interactions, the patient finally opened up about the root cause of his self-injurious behavior, stating that he is chronically plagued by a strong, uncomfortable feeling that he does not really exist. This phenomenon, termed "de-realization," has compelled Conor to injure himself, as the pain and the bleeding that he induced were incontrovertible proof of his existence. Unfortunately, the intense de-realization feeling always eventually returned, and he needed to repeat the behavior again to feel real.

Reflections on the Case

Factitial dermatitis must be distinguished from neurotic excoriations. The main distinction, in terms of the physical aspect, is in how the skin lesions were created. In neurotic excoriations the skin lesions were created by scratching, whereas patients with factitial dermatitis use much more elaborate means of creating skin lesions than simple scratching with their fingernails. These methods include the use of a sharp object such as a knife, injecting chemicals or feces into the skin, and burning the skin with lighted cigarette buds, etc. In terms of the underlying psychopathology, more so than patients with neurotic excoriations, patients with factitial dermatitis frequently experiences intense feelings (e.g., depression, anxiety, stress, etc.) to the point of being bizarre, such as the sensation of de-realization in the above case.

One caveat regarding diagnosing factitial dermatitis is the important distinction between those who are malingering as opposed to those who have true psychopathology. It is an undeniable reality that some patients self-induce bizarre skin lesions for worldly gains, such as disability benefits, insurance payment, getting sympathy or being able to manipulate others. If the factitial dermatitis reflects a conscious and deliberate attempt at these secondary gains, then malingering should be strongly considered. Malingering is not considered a *bona fide* illness either from a physical or psychiatric point-of-view;

thus, no psychiatric diagnosis can be given. In fact, if malingering is conducted for the sake of financial gains such as insurance payment, winning a lawsuit, or for disability payment, such cases actually represent a punishable crime and should be dealt with by law enforcement agencies.

In Conor's case, the factitial dermatitis was created through a motivation that cannot be easily understood by the average person. As such, the case truly represents a psychiatric disorder, and a referral to a psychiatrist is indicated. It is not unusual for him to be initially reluctant to share with you an honest account of how the lesions came about. Direct confrontation is not recommended on your part, since such an approach can make him even more defensive. Typically, as Conor demonstrated, patients with factitial dermatitis tend to come up with rather vague or illogical illness narratives. This phenomenon has been termed the "hollow history."

Since the patient was initially defensive, the authors' recommended approach is to not force the issue but to interact with him in way that conveys your supportive and nonjudgmental attitude. The main goal is to get him to eventually open up about the root cause of his factitial dermatitis and to accept professional help from a psychiatrist or another mental health specialist. In order to achieve this goal, it is critical that you practice highly effective communication and interpersonal skills to establish a good therapeutic rapport with him. In terms of pharmacologic intervention, prescribing medications to improve the pain and prevent infections associated with his ulcerations is appropriate. Patients such as Conor typically recover from factitial dermatitis if they receive psychotherapy and sometimes psycho-pharmacotherapy continuously for a few months from their psychiatrists.

Psychosocial Stressors of Skin Diseases

We have encountered psychocutaneous cases where the psychopathology is the root cause of a patient's skin condition, and the treatment of the underlying psychopathology is essential – sometimes all that is necessary – to resolve his or her cutaneous issues. In this section, we want you to think more broadly about how to address patients whose psychosocial or psychiatric difficulties have chronological relationships with their skin diseases yet no proven causal relationships. For instance, when a patient with psoriasis experiences a new flare coinciding with an inability to tolerate excessive stress, it might be difficult to say for certain that the stress intolerance is directly responsible for the psoriasis flare or vice versa. This type of situations call for a unique term that can encompass both the psychosocial disturbances in the patients' lives and their chronologically associated physiological conditions: *psychophysiological disorders*.

Please refer to Table 24.1 for a list of psychophysiological disorders that are commonly encountered in dermatology.

Psychosomatic and Somatopsychic Aspects of Psychophysiological Disorders

One way to dissect the relationships between psychosocial stressors and skin diseases is to characterize such stressors as either psychosomatic or somatopsychic stressors. The term *psychosomatic* means that external factors contribute to psychological distress, including but not limited to the patients' life world problems, and play a major role in exacerbating their skin conditions, which can be emerging or pre-existing. On the other hand, the term *somatopsychic* refers to the persistent worsening of the skin conditions that by itself has become a psychological difficulty for your patients. Patients getting upset in the dermatology clinic while describing to you how much their skin diseases are bothering them is a good example of the somatopsychic aspect of the psychophysiological disorders.

Psychosomatic and somatopsychic stressors can create a vicious cycle for psychocutaneous disorders, and we hope to illustrate this in the following three cases. Our primary objectives are: (1) to help you become more competent in recognizing and handling psychophysiological disorders in general, and (2) to assist you in formulating treatment plans that can effectively break down the aforementioned vicious cycle.

Chapter 24
Hyperhidrosis and an Anxiety Disorder

Mr. Lewinsky is a 29 year-old man suffering from excessive sweating for as long as he can remember. The patient's general practitioner diagnosed the condition as chronic hyperhidrosis when he was 15. Ever since, he has been treated with several topical drying agents without any benefits. He reports experiencing daily episodes of sweat dripping uncontrollably down his face, palms, and soles. During psychiatric evaluation, he revealed a history of untreated anxiety attacks, which have a temporal relationship with the sweating episodes. The patient disclosed that he had been held at gunpoint in an armed mugging 1 year before the anxiety episodes and uncontrollable sweating began. Any sign of potential danger can trigger the same fear and panic that he experienced during the armed mugging incident.

The decision to start the patient on a benzodiazepine called alprazolam was made. Following a trial of this medication, Mr. Lewinsky's anxiety attacks occurred less frequently and were milder in nature, as were the severity of his concurrent hyperhidrosis episodes. As the residual anxiety attacks and hyperhidrosis episodes persisted, you added another medication, a TCA called doxepin, to the treatment regimen. After 6 months of the combination

T.V. Nguyen et al., *Clinical Cases in Psychocutaneous Disease*, 99
Clinical Cases in Dermatology,
DOI 10.1007/978-1-4471-4312-3_24, © Springer-Verlag London 2014

therapy, the patient was symptom-free. He also began working with a psychotherapist on developing awareness of upcoming anxiety attacks and anxiety-relieving techniques. Another 6 months later, he felt confident enough to make a joint decision with you to begin tapering off alprazolam first and then doxepin in a very gradual, cautious fashion. According to the latest follow-up report, his anxiety disorder and hyperhidrosis are still under control.

Reflections on the Case

It appears that Mr. Lewinsky has an anxiety disorder called post-traumatic stress disorder (PTSD). Based on the context in which his excessive sweating episodes occurred – often when he experienced an episode of his PTSD – the patient's hyperhidrosis can be thought of as one of two things: a primary sweat gland disease made worse/noticeable by his anxiety attacks, or an abnormal manifestation of his physiologic response to the fear element of the anxiety attacks (Table 24.1). There are other subjective and physiological symptoms of anxiety (Table 24.2) in addition to excessive sweating, so please be sure to take a very thorough medical history.

TABLE 24.1 Common psychophysiological disorders in dermatology

Atopic dermatitis
Dyshidrotic eczema
Nummular eczema
Rosacea
Acne
Urticaria
Psoriasis
Neurodermatitis
Pruritus ani

TABLE 24.2 Subjective and physiological symptoms of anxiety

Subjective	Physiological
Stress	Muscle tension
Tension	Shortness of breath
Agitation	Palpitations
Inability to relax	Sweating not due to exertion or exercise
	Frequent urination not due to increased fluid intake

Hyperhidrosis as a stand-alone condition is difficult to control. This patient represents a unique case, where conventional dermatologic therapy may provide very limited benefit. The anxiety disorder component needs to be adequately treated, if the patient is to have any chance at reducing his excessive sweating.

Teaching Points

There are two approaches to managing an anxiety disorder, one is pharmacotherapy, and the other is behavioral psychotherapy, and they are not mutually exclusive. Behavioral psychotherapy consists of strategies to increase awareness of the anxiety attacks and effective relaxation exercises, tailored to each individual's lifestyle and interests. In addition, non-conventional practices such as hypnotism and imagery may be suitable for some patients. Generally, behavioral psychotherapy is almost only reserved for patients who are psychologically minded and in many cases are less effective as monotherapy than in combination with pharmacotherapy.

Anti-anxiety medications consist of two classes: quick-acting benzodiazepines that can be sedating and potentially dependency-causing, and slow-acting benzodiazepines that are not sedating or dependence-inducing. Among quick-acting benzodiazepines, alprazolam is preferred over older agents, such as diazepam and chlordiazepoxide, because its half-life is relatively short and its metabolism is predictable.

With diazepam and chlordiazepoxide, long-term use can result in accumulation of the drugs as well as their active metabolites, leading to a lethargic state that can be bothersome to many patients and their families.

Due to its short half-life, alprazolam is largely eliminated from the patient's body before he or she takes the next dose. As such, the process of tapering off this medication must occur gradually, much similar to slow tapering of oral corticosteroids. Abrupt cessation of the therapeutic effects of alprazolam may lead to a recurrence of the anxiety symptoms. As a result, an inexperienced practitioner may mistake this recurrence for a sign of drug dependence.

Alprazolam comes in various strengths, but the dosages most commonly used in the dermatology practice are 0.25, 0.5, and 1 mg scored tablets. A rule of thumb is to start the patient with a very low dose and carefully titrate the medication up to the optimal dose that can reduce the anxiety without causing sedative side effects. For instance, the practitioner may want to advise the patient to break the 0.25 mg tablets in half and take each 0.125 mg half-tablet four times per day. If the anxiety attacks are not situational but part of a chronic disorder such as PTSD, then the dosage may be increased over a long period of time. Alprazolam should not be prescribed to patients with a history of addiction to the medication. As a drug class warning for all benzodiazepines, patients should be advised to avoid alcoholic beverages while taking alprazolam.

Chapter 25
Atopic Dermatitis and a Major Depressive Disorder

Ms. Reed is a 45 year-old woman with a history of chronic atopic dermatitis, which started when she was in college. At first, she reportedly experienced episodes of patchy, itchy red bumps on the extensor aspects of her arms, legs, and such episodes would get worse during exam periods. After college, she had ten blissful years without any significant atopic dermatitis episodes. However, the disease has been making a return in the past 12–13 years, gradually at first but then picking up speed in terms of frequency and viciousness of each episode. Today, the patient comes in with both arms and legs studded circumferentially with eczematous papules, which appear beefy red and noticeably warm to the touch. She reports still using her triamcinolone acetonide 0.1 % cream and emollients to the affected areas daily. You have never observed such inflammatory intensity with her skin disease before.

When you take a step back to appreciate her overall mood and mannerism, she appears out of the ordinary. Her speech is delayed, as is her comprehension of simple language from you. She admits to feeling tired for the past month and being unable to fall asleep, even at night. You ask if she has lost weight, to which she answers, "I'm not sure, but I don't have much of an appetite these days." "And," she adds, "my mood fluctuates a lot throughout a normal, uneventful day. Sometimes I get really sad and cry for no reason, and all of a sudden, I can just feel okay." You wonder if this patient is depressed, based on her presenting signs and symptoms. Upon further questioning, Ms. Reed tells you that her husband is out of work, which makes things much worse at home because they have had marital problems for several years, and financial stability was the only thing keeping their family together. She is now visibly crying, and you reach for facial tissues to offer her.

Reflections on the Case

According to the Diagnostic and Statistical Manual of Mental Disorders-IV (DSM-IV), our patient meets the criteria for a major depressive episode (MDE). The psychosomatic and somatopsychic manifestations of her depression exacerbated and perpetuate her atopic dermatitis, rendering it resistant to conventional dermatologic therapy that would have otherwise been efficacious. She can benefit from a combination of psychopharmacologic therapy, behavioral psychotherapy, and dermatologic treatment.

You should write her for an anti-depressant with a sedative and anti-pruritic effect, such as doxepin, and an anti-anxiety agent, such as alprazolam. The alprazolam will help with any acute anxiety episodes she might have, as she is experiencing significant stress from her financial and marital strain. Additionally, its sedative property might be a nice "side effect" for this patient, who has not been able to have a normal sleep cycle. A referral to a behavioral modification expert, such as a psychologist, should be made to reduce her scratching, which worsens the atopic dermatitis. Such control of behavior can be achieved with exercises such as keeping the patient's hands in her pockets whenever she feels the urge to scratch or squeezing a stress ball with her free hands

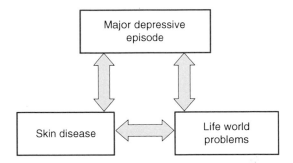

FIGURE 25.1 The vicious cycle of atopic dermatitis and a major depressive disorder. The *arrows* represent reciprocal relationships among the three major factors contributing to the patient's psychophysiological disorder

until the urge passes. You instruct Ms. Reed to continue her topical steroid treatment with liberal use of emollients; plus, you give her a new prescription for a topical antibiotic ointment to reduce bacterial colonization, and consequentially, the risk of skin infections.

Teaching Points

The patient's current MDE is likely to be a result of her life world problems and may have contributed to worsening of her atopic dermatitis. In addition, the recalcitrant atopic dermatitis might be a somatopsychic aspect of her psychophysiological disorder. Keep in mind that no matter how you conceptualize her disease, all three factors of her psychophysiological disorder (the patient's MDE, skin issues, and life world problems) form a vicious cycle and need to be targeted separately for optimal outcomes (Fig. 25.1).

Table 25.1 contains information from the DSM-IV that may assist you in making the diagnosis of a "major depressive episode," which is the terminology used by mental health professions to distinguish serious cases of depression that can benefit from pharmacologic therapy from less serious cases casually referred to as "depression." You only need to identify a total of five symptoms to make the diagnosis; however,

TABLE 25.1 Subjective and physiological symptoms of a major depressive episode (MDE)

Subjective symptoms	Physiologic symptoms
Depressed mood (with or without crying spells)	Fatigue
Anhedonia	Insomnia (night)
Excessive guilt	Hypersomnia (day)
Helplessness	Appetite disturbances
Hopelessness	Inattention
Worthlessness	Memory deficit
Suicidal ideation	Psychomotor agitation or retardation
	Constipation

both subjective and physiologic symptoms must be present in order for the episode to quality as an MDE.

The subjective symptoms of an MDE include seemingly unprovoked crying or mourning, persistently depressed mood, anhedonia (the inability to feel pleasure from activities that produce pleasure normally), excessive guilt, hopelessness, helplessness, and feeling worthless. The physiological symptoms of an MDE range from altered sleep patterns (night-time insomnia and daytime hypersomnia), altered appetite or eating habits (low appetite, no appetite, or too much appetite resulting in hyperphagia), inability to concentrate, memory deficit, fatigue, altered psychomotor activity (agitation or retardation), and constipation. Patients can be sub-classified as having "agitated" depression, where they become restless and easily hostile when provoked, or "retarded" depression, where they show lack of energy and slowed speech, mentation, etc. Many patients with neurotic excoriations due to depression or those experiencing exacerbation of chronic skin inflammation as a result of an MDE belong to the "agitated" sub-class.

When attempting to diagnose depression, you should be aware that some patients deny feeling depressed, despite showing sadness and even tearfulness. This is perhaps due to the social stigma associated with such a diagnosis or the fact that such patients use denial as a coping mechanism. If you encounter a patient who denies what you truly think is an MDE, please do not confront the patient. Avoid getting into an argument with your patients in generally, but such advice is especially important in sensitive situations such as this. Without good rapport, it will be difficult to get the patient to accept behavioral psychotherapy or psychopharmacologic therapy.

It may be more helpful to focus on eliciting physiological symptoms of major depression, including sleep and appetite changes. Toward this end, we prefer the aforementioned approach, whereby the patient feels as if the questions are part of routine questioning about her general medical condition. Next, you should ask the patient "how is everything else in your life?" to provide an avenue for her to discuss life world problems. After having done this, the patient may realize that her interpersonal relationship issues played a part in creating her psychological difficulties, and as a consequence, you may be one step closer to gaining her cooperation.

With regard to using doxepin to control the patient's current condition, please keep in mind that it has a similar side effect profile to the other older TCAs, including disturbance of cardiac conduction, weight gain, orthostatic hypotension, and anti-cholinergic effects. Prolonged QT intervals, which can be documented as part of the EKG test, can lead to serious cardiac adverse events. Please follow the latest guidelines to ensure proper administration and monitoring of this drug. Generally, patients who are known to have cardiac conduction disturbances or geriatric patients must obtain a baseline EKG test before starting treatment. If rhythm abnormalities exist, the patient might not be a suitable candidate for doxepin.

New anti-depressive agents (e.g., fluoxetine, sertraline, paroxetine, etc.) are SSRIs, and thus should be free of the side effects associated with doxepin and other TCAs. It is more convenient to titrate them because fewer steps are required to reach the therapeutic dose. Since cardiac conduction is not affected, they are often safe to use in geriatric patients and those with a history of cardiac conduction disturbances. However, they have a different adverse effect profile, including reduced sexual drive, erectile dysfunction, nausea, diarrhea, insomnia, etc.

Chapter 26
Psoriasis and Excessive Stress

Erica is a 19-year-old college student, who presented with a severe flare of her chronic plaque-type psoriasis. She describes the lesions as being very pruritic, to the point where she needs to take anti-allergy medication at night in order to fall asleep. The patient worries that she will fail her final examinations coming up next month in English Literature and Evolutionary Biology, two rather challenging courses. Despite tireless efforts to prepare for the exams, her self-assessment tests predict that she will score in the bottom half of each respective class, which is causing her significant distress. In addition, she is the captain of the cheerleading team at her university, and her responsibilities have doubled in the past few weeks due to her co-captain dropping out of the program.

While sharing her difficulties with you, Erica struggles to fight back tears. She is the oldest of three sisters and feels pressured to keep up with her family's expectation that she remains a role model for her younger siblings. However, her self-confidence is waning as the amounts of work and stress are mounting. Physical exam reveals well demarcated, "beefy red" erythematous plaques with thick micaceous scales symmetrically scattered over the arms, legs, backs, and buttocks. There is noticeable dried blood on the plaques on her shins,

T.V. Nguyen et al., *Clinical Cases in Psychocutaneous Disease*, 109
Clinical Cases in Dermatology,
DOI 10.1007/978-1-4471-4312-3_26, © Springer-Verlag London 2014

where Erica reports that she scratches repeatedly to relieve the severe itch.

Previously, the patient has applied high-potency topical steroids and taken short courses of methotrexate to control similarly severe psoriasis flares. In between these flares, her psoriasis was successfully treated with a combination of a mid-potency topical steroid and calcipotriene cream. Erica has read on the Internet that methotrexate and other systemic medications will damage her internal organs if used too many times. Therefore, she requests you to not prescribe any systemic medications today. She is not a candidate for phototherapy because of her hectic schedule. In consideration of her request and the stressful circumstances surrounding her current psoriasis flare, you suggest trial of a combination of psychological therapy and high-potency topical steroids for 4 weeks. She accepts this experimental treatment and asks for a referral to a psychologist.

Two weeks later, you see Erica back in your office. The patient states that she enjoys seeing her psychologist very much, and the psychologist has helped her work out many of her issues. As a result of regular counseling sessions thrice weekly, and application of the topical steroid daily for 2 weeks, her psoriasis has been significantly reduced. You congratulate Erica and ask your receptionist to schedule a follow-up visit in 2 weeks.

Teaching Points

Elucidating the role of psychological stress and understanding how it affects physical ailments can be daunting tasks. Based on chronology, Erica's psoriasis flare appears to be induced or exacerbated by the excessive stress in her personal life. You get to decide whether or not to target this excessive stress. Per Erica's request, your options for conventional dermatologic therapy are limited to topical agents; yet, you know that her current skin condition requires more than topical treatment. There is nothing to lose from combing high-potency topical steroids with stress reduction therapy. If you decided to pursue this route, the extent of your engagement would be limited to making a referral for mental health counseling and following up to make sure that she is benefiting from it.

Working with a Psychiatrist

In addition to patients with psychological difficulties, such as excessive stress or depression, you may encounter patients with true psychiatric conditions (e.g., major depressive disorder, schizophrenia, panic disorder, etc.). Such psychiatric conditions may significantly impair your ability to establish rapport with your patients, and consequently, your ability to treat their skin diseases. This may necessitate a consultation with psychiatry and, depending on the nature of the patient's psychiatric condition, may lead to the use of psychotropic medications at the psychiatrist's discretion. If the patient would like for you to consult a psychiatrist, we hope that you will be prepared to choose and to work well with one. Please keep in mind that there might be opportunities and pitfalls from working with psychiatry. We hope to help you minimize or avoid these pitfalls, if at all possible, via the following discussion.

In general, psychiatrists may subscribe to more than one theory about how to treat psychopathologies, ranging from psychotherapy, hypnosis, and behavioral therapy to psychopharmacotherapy. Those who are extreme enthusiasts of the "psychodynamic" approach tend to believe that psychological conflicts are the root causes of most psychological and psychiatric disorders. According to this school of thought, medications used to normalize the patients' emotional or mental states may cover up true symptoms of their psychopathologies, thus rendering the patients' psychological conflicts difficult to deal with. In addition, psychodynamic therapy enthusiasts tend to distrust psychometric tests used to help psychiatrists diagnose certain psychiatric conditions.

On the opposite end of the spectrum of approaches held by psychiatrists is the viewpoint that psychopathologies stem from biochemical abnormalities in the human brain rather than psychological conflicts. With respect to diagnosing psychiatric conditions, the biologically oriented psychiatrists are generally not shy to employ standardized definitions, including those in the DSM-IV, and quantitative, psychometric tools. In terms of therapy, they frequently favor psychopharmacotherapy as opposed to emotional counseling or psychotherapy to target the biochemical processes that might be responsible for the patients' emotional or cognitive disturbances. This is believed to eventually correct the symptomatology of the patients' psychopathologies, including their psychosocial difficulties.

As a dermatology practitioner, you should be aware of the aforementioned extreme viewpoints, their derivative approaches to the treatment of psychopathologies, and everything in between. More importantly, please keep in mind that despite our best intentions to help our patients, most (if not all) dermatologists are limited in our capacity to diagnose and treat psychiatric problems. Hence, it is necessary to select psychiatrists who are willing to be flexible in helping you take care of the psychodermatology patients' problems. You and your patients may benefit more from such psychiatric consultants than those with recommendations that are vague, speculative, or full of psychiatry jargon without any adequate explanations.

Patients with psychocutaneous disorders seldom seek help from psychiatry for two reasons. One, such patients may be in denial of the psychopathologies associated with their dermatologic conditions. Two, even if they are aware of the need to see a psychiatry practitioner, the social stigma associated with seeking psychiatric help (e.g., being labeled "crazy") frequently causes them to hesitate. As a consequence of these factors, you may encounter psychiatric consultants with excellent reputations within their field yet limited knowledge or experience with psychocutaneous cases. Or, it may be that their definitions of what constitute psychiatric diagnoses are different from yours. Your referral documents should contain adequate background information about the nature of the psychodermatological diagnosis plus specific objectives of the treatment plan that you would like the psychiatrist to help you accomplish. There might be things that he or she is unfamiliar with or considers outdated, so be ready to defend your choices using the literature related to psychodermatology. One example is the use of pimozide, which in psychiatry has largely been replaced with newer anti-psychotic medications.

It is helpful to introduce the psychiatry practitioner to the patient as a member of your team. This acknowledgement may ease the patient into establishing a relationship with the consultant without feeling abandoned by you. There might be special circumstances where the psychiatric consultants are so kind as to agree to see the patient in the dermatologic clinic. This is not to be expected on a regular basis, so please think carefully before selecting the patients and the cases for which to make such a special request. Again, having a flexible, accommodating psychiatric consultant will make your life easier, and in the end will benefit your patients tremendously.

References

1. Levinson W, Roter DL, Mullooly JP, Dull VT, Frankel RM. Physician-patient communication. The relationship with malpractice claims among primary care physicians and surgeons. JAMA. 1997;277(7):553–9.
2. Hickson GB, Clayton EW, Githens PB, Sloan FA. Factors that prompted families to file medical malpractice claims following perinatal injuries. JAMA. 1992;267(10):1359–63.
3. Vincent C, Young M, Phillips A. Why do people sue doctors? A study of patients and relatives taking legal action. Lancet. 1994;343(8913):1609–13.
4. Brenner RJ, Bartholomew L. Communication errors in radiology: a liability cost analysis. J Am Coll Radiol. 2005;2(5):428–31.
5. Renzi C, Picardi A, Abeni D, et al. Association of dissatisfaction with care and psychiatric morbidity with poor treatment compliance. Arch Dermatol. 2002;138(3):337–42.
6. Forster HP, Schwartz J, DeRenzo E. Reducing legal risk by practicing patient-centered medicine. Arch Intern Med. 2002;162(11): 1217–9.
7. Uhlenhake EE, Kurkowski D, Feldman SR. Conversations on psoriasis–what patients want and what physicians can provide: a qualitative look at patient and physician expectations. J Dermatolog Treat. 2010;21(1):6–12.
8. Jackson SA. The epidemiology of aging. In: Hazzard WR, Blass JP, Ettinger WHJ, Halter JB, Ouslander JG, editors. Principles of geriatric medicine and gerontology. 4th ed. New York: McGraw-Hill; 1999. p. 203–25.
9. Kinsella K, He W. Census Bureau, international population reports, P95/09-1, an aging world: 2008. Washington, DC: U.S. Government Printing Office; 2009.

116   References

10. Wykoff RF. Delusions of parasitosis: a review. Rev Infect Dis. 1987;9(3):433–7.
11. Skott A. Delusions of infestation. Reports from the psychiatric research center. No. 13. Göteborg: St. Jörgen's Hospital, University of Göteborg; 1978.
12. Wilson JW, Miller HE. Delusion of parasitosis (acarophobia). Arch Derm Syphilol. 1946;54:39–56.
13. Koo J, Lee CS. Delusions of parasitosis. A dermatologist's guide to diagnosis and treatment. Am J Clin Dermatol. 2001;2(5):285–90.
14. Koo J. Psychodermatology: a practical manual for clinicians. Curr Probl Dermatol. 1995;7(6):204–32.
15. Koblenzer CS. Psychocutaneous disease. 1st ed. Orlando: Grune and Stratton; 1987.
16. Michelson HE. Psychosomatic studies in dermatology: the motivation of self-induced eruptions. Arch Dermatol. 1945;51(4):245–50.
17. Zaidens SH. Self-inflicted dermatoses and their psychodynamics. J Nerv Ment Dis. 1951;113(5):395–404.
18. Heller MM, Koo JYM. Neurotic excoriations, acne excoriee, and factitial dermatitis. In: Heller MM, Koo JYM, editors. Contemporary diagnosis and management in psychodermatology. 1st ed. Newton: Handbooks in Health Care Co; 2011. p. 37–44.
19. Koblenzer CS. Psychiatric syndromes of interest to dermatologists. Int J Dermatol. 1993;32(2):82–8.
20. Jermain DM, Crismon ML. Pharmacotherapy of obsessive-compulsive disorder. Pharmacotherapy. 1990;10(3):175–98.
21. Koblenzer CS. Pharmacology of psychotropic drugs useful in dermatologic practice. Int J Dermatol. 1993;32(3):162–8.
22. Koblenzer CS, Bostrom P. Chronic cutaneous dysesthesia syndrome: a psychotic phenomenon or a depressive symptom? J Am Acad Dermatol. 1994;30(2 Pt 2):370–4.
23. Brewer JD, Meves A, Bostwick JM, Hamacher KL, Pittelkow MR. Cocaine abuse: dermatologic manifestations and therapeutic approaches. J Am Acad Dermatol. 2008;59(3):483–7.
24. Elpern DJ. Cocaine abuse and delusions of parasitosis. Cutis. 1988;42(4):273–4.
25. Bach M, Bach D. Psychiatric and psychometric issues in acne excoriee. Psychother Psychosom. 1993;60(3–4):207–10.
26. Arnold LM, Auchenbach MB, McElroy SL. Psychogenic excoriation. Clinical features, proposed diagnostic criteria, epidemiology and approaches to treatment. CNS Drugs. 2001;15(5):351–9.

27. Shah KN, Fried RG. Factitial dermatoses in children. Curr Opin Pediatr. 2006;18(4):403–9.

28. Arnold LM, McElroy SL, Mutasim DF, Dwight MM, Lamerson CL, Morris EM. Characteristics of 34 adults with psychogenic excoriation. J Clin Psychiatry. 1998;59(10):509–14.

29. Wilhelm S, Keuthen NJ, Deckersbach T, et al. Self-injurious skin picking: clinical characteristics and comorbidity. J Clin Psychiatry. 1999;60(7):454–9.

30. McElroy SL, Phillips KA, Keck Jr PE. Obsessive compulsive spectrum disorder. J Clin Psychiatry. 1994;55(Suppl):33–51. discussion 52–33.

31. Oldham JM, Phillips KA, Skodol AE. Impulsivity and compulsivity. Washington, DC: American Psychiatric Press; 1996.

32. Koo J, Lee CS. Psychocutaneous medicine. New York: Marcel Dekker; 2003.

33. Simeon D, Stein DJ, Gross S, Islam N, Schmeidler J, Hollander E. A double-blind trial of fluoxetine in pathologic skin picking. J Clin Psychiatry. 1997;58(8):341–7.

34. Gupta MA, Guptat AK. The use of antidepressant drugs in dermatology. J Eur Acad Dermatol Venereol. 2001;15(6):512–8.

35. Kalivas J, Kalivas L, Gilman D, Hayden CT. Sertraline in the treatment of neurotic excoriations and related disorders. Arch Dermatol. 1996;132(5):589–90.

36. Kearney CA, Silverman WK. Treatment of an adolescent with obsessive-compulsive disorder by alternating response prevention and cognitive therapy: an empirical analysis. J Behav Ther Exp Psychiatry. 1990;21(1):39–47.

37. Mancebo MC, Eisen JL, Sibrava NJ, Dyck IR, Rasmussen SA. Patient utilization of cognitive-behavioral therapy for OCD. Behav Ther. 2011;42(3):399–412.

38. Alster TS, Kurban AK, Grove GL, Grove MJ, Tan OT. Alteration of argon laser-induced scars by the pulsed dye laser. Lasers Surg Med. 1993;13(3):368–73.

39. Bowes LE, Alster TS. Treatment of facial scarring and ulceration resulting from acne excoriee with 585-nm pulsed dye laser irradiation and cognitive psychotherapy. Dermatol Surg. 2004;30(6):934–8.

40. Shenefelt PD. Biofeedback, cognitive-behavioral methods, and hypnosis in dermatology: is it all in your mind? Dermatol Ther. 2003;16(2):114–22.

41. Ratliff RG, Stein NH. Treatment of neurodermatitis by behavior therapy: a case study. Behav Res Ther. 1968;6(3):397–9.
42. Rosenbaum MS, Ayllon T. The behavioral treatment of neurodermatitis through habit-reversal. Behav Res Ther. 1981;19(4):313–8.
43. Kent A, Drummond LM. Acne excoriee–a case report of treatment using habit reversal. Clin Exp Dermatol. 1989;14(2):163–4.

Index

Printed by Publishers' Graphics LLC